# Preventive Medicine
# and
# Public Health

*1st Edition*

D0207412

A USMLE STEP 2 REVIEW

# Preventive Medicine and Public Health

## 1st Edition

# 700

## Questions & Answers

**Richard H. Hart, MD, DrPH**
*Dean, School of Public Health*
*Chair, Department of Preventive Medicine*
*School of Medicine*
*Loma Linda University*
*Loma Linda, California*

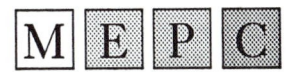

APPLETON & LANGE
Stamford, Connecticut

Copyright © 1996 by Appleton & Lange
A Simon & Schuster Company
© 1991 by Elsevier Science Publishing Co., Inc.

All rights reserved. This book, or any parts thereof, may not be used or reproduced in any manner without written permission. For information, address Appleton & Lange, Four Stamford Plaza, PO Box 120041, Stamford, Connecticut 06912-0041.

96  97  98  99  /  10  9  8  7  6  5  4  3  2  1

Prentice Hall International (UK) Limited, *London*
Prentice Hall of Australia Pty. Limited, *Sydney*
Prentice Hall Canada. Inc., *Toronto*
Prentice Hall Hispanoamericana. S.A., *Mexico*
Prentice Hall of India Private Limited, *New Delhi*
Prentice Hall of Japan, Inc., *Tokyo*
Simon & Schuster Asia Pte. Ltd., *Singapore*
Editora Prentice Hall do Brasil Ltda., *Rio de Janeiro*
Prentice Hall, *Upper Saddle River, New Jersey*

ISBN  0-8385-6319-8

90000

9 780838 563199

ISBN: 0–8385–6319–8
ISSN: 1086–7562

*Acquisitions Editor*: Marinita Timban
*Production Editor*: Jeanmarie M. Roche
*Designer*: Mary Skudlarek

PRINTED IN THE UNITED STATES OF AMERICA

# Contents

# CONTRIBUTORS

David J. Berglund, MD
Preventive Medicine Resident
Loma Linda University

J. Xavier Castillo, MD
Preventive Medicine Resident
Loma Linda University

David T. Dyjack, CIH, MSPH
Chair and Assistant Professor of Environmental and Occupational Health
Loma Linda University School of Public Health

Linda H. Ferry, MD, MPH
Program Director
Preventive Medicine Residency and
    Assistant Professor of Health Promotion and Education
Loma Linda University School of Public Health

Kenneth W. Hart, MD, MPH
Assistant Professor of International Health
Loma Linda University School of Public Health

Richard H. Hart, MD, DrPH
Dean
School of Public Health and
Chair
Department of Public Health and Preventive Medicine
School of Medicine
Loma Linda University

Ronald P. Hattis, MD, MPH
Associate Clinical Professor of Health Administration
Loma Linda University School of Public Health

Calvin G. Huey, MD
Preventive Medicine Resident
Loma Linda University

Holly A. Jason, MD
Preventive Medicine Resident
Loma Linda University

John Morgan, DrPH
Associate Professor of Epidemiology and Biostatistics
Loma Linda University School of Public Health

Eric Ngo, MD, MPH
Associate Clinical Professor of Health Promotion and Education
Loma Linda University School of Public Health

J. Rochelle Parker, MD
Preventive Medicine Resident
Loma Linda University

Vivian Pereyra, MD, MPH
Preventive Medicine Resident
Loma Linda University

Minal M. Patel, MBBcH, MPH
Preventive Medicine Resident
Loma Linda University

Warren R. Peters, MD
Director, Center for Health Promotion
Assistant Professor of Health Promotion and Education
Loma Linda University School of Public Health

Thomas J. Prendergast, MD, MPH
Associate Clinical Professor of Epidemiology and Biostatistics
Loma Linda University School of Public Health

Pamela A. Sieler, MD
Preventive Medicine Resident
Loma Linda University

Gwendolyn D. Taylor-Holmes, MD, JD
Preventive Medicine Resident
Loma Linda University

Susan H. Yandle, MD, MPH
Preventive Medicine Resident
Loma Linda University

# Preface

For many medical students the disciplines of public health and preventive medicine have seemed to be a necessary evil on their way to a clinical career. Subjects such as statistics, epidemiology, environmental health, and health care organization were all learned to pass examinations and then often stored in irretrievable memory. In today's health care climate, however, population-based issues are of increasing importance, with the requirements of managed care making it essential for all practicing physicians to have an understanding of underlying principles.

The questions and answers in this book are designed to introduce you to the core concepts of public health. They are written specifically to address the level of concerns contained in the USMLE Step 2 examination. A combination of content areas, disease control issues, and organizational concerns provides coverage of the broad discipline of public health. Each reader is encouraged to make an honest struggle with the question before reviewing the explanation. Additional reading is listed in the reference cited for each question.

As the financial impact of health care reform causes continued ripples through our system, it becomes increasingly important for each of us to learn new styles of practicing medicine. Population-based issues will gain increasing prominence as a method of obtaining cost efficiency in our care of patients. Our hope is that review of this material will not only help with examinations but will also provide a foundation of understanding that will be valuable in your future career.

**Richard H. Hart, MD, DrPH**

# 1

# Public Health Methods

---

**DIRECTIONS:** Each of the numbered items or incomplete statements in this section is followed by answers or completions of the statement. Select the **ONE** lettered answer or completion that is **BEST** in each case.

---

1. A child aged 2 years is being seen for a well-child checkup. Which of the following is a leading potential cause of death for this child for which a preventive measure is available and which should be addressed with the parents?
   A. Lead toxicity
   B. Motor vehicle accident
   C. Tuberculosis
   D. Pneumonia
   E. Influenza

2. For a man aged 40 to 50 years with no known medical problems, which of the following screening tests should routinely be performed?
   A. Urinalysis
   B. Sigmoidoscopy
   C. Cholesterol
   D. Prostate specific antigen
   E. None of the above

3. A slender 50-year-old white woman with fair skin is being seen for a routine Papanicolaou (Pap) smear. She is postmenopausal and in good health with no known medical problems. Her activity level is sedentary, and she spends most of her time indoors. Which of the following preventive measures would be most appropriate for her?
   A. Electrocardiogram
   B. Discussion of aspirin therapy
   C. Discussion of estrogen replacement therapy
   D. Instruction to use skin protection from UV light
   E. None of the above

4. Treatment of a person with AIDS using AZT is what level of prevention?
   A. Primary prevention
   B. Secondary prevention
   C. Tertiary prevention
   D. All of the above
   E. None of the above

5. Treatment of a person with AIDS using trimethoprim-sulfamethoxazole is what level of prevention?
   A. Primary prevention
   B. Secondary prevention
   C. Tertiary prevention
   D. All of the above
   E. None of the above

6. Successful treatment of *Pneumocystis carinii* pneumonia in an HIV-positive patient will
   A. increase the prevalence of AIDS by increasing the incidence of AIDS
   B. increase the prevalence of AIDS by increasing the duration of AIDS
   C. not alter the prevalence of HIV in the community
   D. represent a form of tertiary prevention of *P. carinii* pneumonia
   E. increase the incidence of AIDS

**7.** The risk of acquiring hepatitis A is measured by
  **A.** the incidence times the average duration of hepatitis A
  **B.** the number of existing cases divided by the duration of hepatitis A
  **C.** the incidence of hepatitis A
  **D.** the number of new cases of hepatitis A
  **E.** the number of existing cases divided by the population at risk

### Questions 8–10:

In a community of 100,000 persons, there were 1000 existing cases of disease X at the beginning of 1993. During 1993, 100 new cases of this disease were diagnosed, while 500 persons died of disease X during the year. Assume that disease X is a nonrepeating chronic illness. Match the following:

**8.** The annual prevalence of disease X for this population during 1993 was
  **A.** 75 per 100,000
  **B.** 101 per 100,000
  **C.** 500 per 100,000
  **D.** 1000 per 100,000
  **E.** 1100 per 100,000

**9.** The risk for disease X for this population during 1993 was
  **A.** 75 per 100,000
  **B.** 101 per 100,000
  **C.** 500 per 100,000
  **D.** 1000 per 100,000
  **E.** 1100 per 100,000

**10.** The risk of death from disease X for this population during 1993 was
  **A.** 75 per 100,000
  **B.** 101 per 100,000
  **C.** 500 per 100,000
  **D.** 1000 per 100,000
  **E.** 1100 per 100,000

**Questions 11–14:**
Match the following. Each choice may be used only once:

    **A.** infectivity
    **B.** pathogenicity
    **C.** viability
    **D.** virulence

**11.** The propensity for *Neisseria meningitides* to produce severe and fatal disease.

**12.** The capacity of the HIV virus to survive in a defined environment outside the human body.

**13.** The capacity of the influenza virus to enter, survive and multiply inside a host.

**14.** The capacity of toxigenic *Escherichia coli* to produce the functional, morphologic, and pathologic changes that cause symptomatic disease.

**15.** An example of fomite transmission of a disease-producing agent is transmission from
    **A.** clothing contaminated by body lice
    **B.** dust particles contaminated by rhinovirus
    **C.** mountain spring water contaminated by *Giardia*
    **D.** bite of mosquito infected by *Plasmodium vivax*
    **E.** food contaminated by *Staphylococcus*

**Questions 16–19:**
Match the following.

    **A.** cross-sectional
    **B.** case–control
    **C.** ecologic
    **D.** cohort

**16.** An investigation that evaluated the association between the incidence of pancreatic cancer and the per capita sales of beef in 30 South American countries.

17. A research team follows 1200 HIV positive patients at an outpatient clinic over 3 years to determine the incidence of cerebral toxoplasmosis.

18. Urine samples were collected from 29,000 pregnant women admitted for delivery to 202 hospitals throughout the state for determination of maternal alcohol and drug use at the time of the infants' delivery.

19. Medical records of 73 people with hepatitis B were reviewed to determine if there is an association between their previous vaccination status and their chances of contracting hepatitis B.

20. Specificity is
    A. the probability that a person with latent syphilis will have a reactive RPR
    B. the probability that a person without syphilis will have a reactive RPR
    C. the probability that a person without syphilis will have a nonreactive RPR
    D. the probability that a person with syphilis has a false positive RPR
    E. the probability that a person with syphilis has a reactive RPR

21. The crude birth rate, the most fundamental fertility measure, uses
    A. all births in the numerator and total population in the denominator
    B. all births in the numerator and women 15 to 44 years of age in the denominator
    C. the sum of all of the age-specific fertility rates by single years of age
    D. births to women in a specific age range in the numerator
    E. total fertility rate minus crude death rate

22. Fertility refers to
    A. the capacity to bear children
    B. the probability of conceiving in a given month
    C. the actual birth of living offspring
    D. the probability of conceiving in a given year per 1000 women
    E. ratio of live births to total pregnancies

23. The country with the highest life expectancy at birth for males, reaching 75.5 years in 1986, is
    A. Canada
    B. United States
    C. Japan
    D. Sweden
    E. Germany

24. As we near the year 2000, what percentage of the world's population is found in urban areas?
    A. 22%
    B. 40%
    C. 60%
    D. 75%
    E. 80%

25. The main reason that population growth rates in lesser developed countries have accelerated during the past several generations is
    A. birth rates have increased in rural areas
    B. death rates have decreased
    C. death rates have remained steady as a result of better living conditions
    D. a result of high fertility rates
    E. a result of a drop in both birth and death rates

26. A country with a rapidly growing population has the following characteristic
    A. 40% to 50% of the population is less than 15 years of age
    B. a crude birth rate of 20 to 30
    C. high doubling time
    D. a low migration rate
    E. economic stability

27. If a country has a crude birth rate of 35 per 1000 people per year and a crude death rate of 15 per 1000 per year, what is its growth rate?
    A. 20%
    B. 2%
    C. 2.3%
    D. 5%
    E. 7%

**28.** The majority of the known cases of hantavirus transmission have occurred by which mode in the United States?
  **A.** Laboratory exposure
  **B.** Fecal-oral
  **C.** Inhalation of aerosols
  **D.** Intimate contact
  **E.** Arthropod bites

**29.** All of the following are practical preventive measures against infection by *Cryptosporidium* during a community water-borne outbreak, **EXCEPT**
  **A.** maintaining strict hand washing
  **B.** avoidance of swimming in public pools
  **C.** chlorination of public potable water supply
  **D.** practice of safer sex
  **E.** control of fecal-oral transmission

**30.** Assume that surveillance for a specific disease has been implemented and that an appropriate screening test is being sought. Which of the following is most important for an effective surveillance system screening test?
  **A.** High complexity
  **B.** High specificity
  **C.** High predictive value positive
  **D.** Low predictive value negative
  **E.** Low flexibility

**31.** Data from which of the following types of records would allow for evaluation of incidence of a specific type of cancer in a geographic region?
  **A.** Disease case registry
  **B.** Population-based registry
  **C.** Review of hospital records
  **D.** Review of mortality records
  **E.** None of the above

32. In an ongoing epidemic the health department may initiate active surveillance by directly contacting clinicians for current information. Regarding the data obtained and cases detected, which of the following will be increased by this active surveillance?
   A. Sensitivity
   B. Specificity
   C. Representativeness
   D. Predictive value positive
   E. None of the above

33. In an epidemiologic investigation of an outbreak of cases of unknown origin (or an epidemic), which of the following should have highest priority?
   A. Confirmation of the diagnosis for cases
   B. Verification of the existence of an epidemic
   C. Development and testing of an explanatory hypothesis
   D. Proposal of measures for control of the health problem
   E. Search for additional cases of the suspect disease

34. An observational study examined 649 cases of lung cancer, finding 647 of them to have a history of smoking. Of 649 controls, there were 622 who had a past history of smoking. The incidence of lung cancer among smokers (or risk of lung cancer among smokers) may be calculated as follows
   A. $647/(647 + 622)$
   B. $(647 \times 27)/(2 \times 622)$
   C. $647/649$
   D. $2/649$
   E. Cannot be calculated using the data given

35. For which of the following would a case–control study generally be advantageous, as opposed to a cohort study or other study?
   A. A study of a common, acute disease
   B. A study of a rare disease, with long latency
   C. A study to determine multiple effects from a single exposure
   D. A study to elucidate the mechanism of disease
   E. A study to ascertain the effects of treatment for a disease

**36.** A cohort study of a measles outbreak in a school obtained the following data:

|  | | Measles | |
|---|---|---|---|
|  | | Present | Absent |
| **Known Exposure at School** | Present | 21 | 453 |
|  | Absent | 49 | 1307 |

How should the relative risk of measles for those with and without known exposure be calculated?
**A.** (21 × 1307) divided by (49 × 453)
**B.** [21/(21 + 453)] divided by [49/(49 + 1307)]
**C.** (21/453) − (49/1307)
**D.** [21/(21 + 453)] − [49/(49 + 1307)]
**E.** Cannot be calculated from the data given

**37.** When a screening test for HIV is performed, an ELISA test is first done and it is repeated if positive. If the second test is positive, a Western blot test is performed for confirmation. Subsequently a p24 antigen test may also be performed. This serial interpretation has which of the following effects?
**A.** Increases both the sensitivity and the specificity
**B.** Increases the predictive value positive and slightly decreases the sensitivity
**C.** Increases the predictive value positive and slightly increases the sensitivity
**D.** Increases both the specificity and the predictive value negative
**E.** Has no effect on the sensitivity or specificity

**38.** A true incidence rate for a specific disease is properly calculated as
   **A.** cases in a population with onset during a specific time period, divided by the population size at the start of the time period
   **B.** cases present in a population during a specific time period, divided by the population size at the start of the time period
   **C.** cases in a population with onset during a specific time period, divided by the sum of the time periods of susceptibility for all the individuals in the population
   **D.** cases present in a population during a specific time period, divided by the product of the population size and the time period of observation
   **E.** cases in a population with onset during a specific time period, divided by the population size at the end of the time period

**39.** Select the correct denominator used for the common computation of the "infant mortality rate."
   **A.** number of deaths among persons aged less than 1 year in a population during a given year
   **B.** number of live births in a population during a year
   **C.** number of person years of infancy for a population during a year
   **D.** number of live births and number of infant deaths for a population during a year
   **E.** number of infants in a population on July 1 of a year

**40.** In which of the following situations would it be preferable to use a hazards rate rather than either cumulative incidence or an incidence rate?
   **A.** The disease is very common
   **B.** The disease is very rare
   **C.** The risk of the disease for the upcoming year must be predicted
   **D.** Disease cases differ from the general population on specific demographic characteristics
   **E.** There is an ongoing outbreak of the disease

41. A ratio of two cumulative incidence proportions is often used to contrast incidence measures. In different studies, different measures may be used to approximate this ratio. Which of the following would *never* be expected to approximate this ratio?
    A. Incidence rate ratio
    B. Hazards rate ratio
    C. Relative risk
    D. Risk difference
    E. Odds ratio

42. Among persons having a specific disease, which of the following measures the risk of death from that disease?
    A. The disease-specific proportion of mortality
    B. The disease-specific case-fatality proportion
    C. The disease-specific mortality proportion
    D. The standardized mortality ratio
    E. The product of the prevalence and the standardized mortality ratio

43. Risk of death from AIDS in the city of San Francisco would best be assessed using which of the following measures?
    A. The AIDS-specific proportion of mortality
    B. The AIDS-specific mortality proportion
    C. The AIDS-specific case-fatality proportion
    D. The relative risk of death for the population with AIDS
    E. The incidence of AIDS in San Francisco

44. Risk of developing AIDS in the city of San Francisco would best be assessed using which of the following measures?
    A. The AIDS-specific proportion of mortality
    B. The AIDS-specific mortality proportion
    C. The AIDS-specific case-fatality proportion
    D. The relative risk of death for the population with AIDS
    E. The incidence of AIDS in San Francisco

**45.** A study in Uganda found a proportional mortality resulting from cancer of 1%. This compares to findings of a proportional mortality from cancer of 6% in the United States. What may be concluded on the basis of the above findings?
  **A.** Relative risk of dying from cancer in the United States compared to Uganda is 6
  **B.** Uganda has a lower prevalence of cancer than the United States
  **C.** A larger proportion of deaths in Uganda may be attributed to causes other than cancer
  **D.** Uganda has a lower cancer-specific mortality rate than the United States
  **E.** More carcinogens are present in the environment in the United States than in Uganda

**46.** Treatment of AIDS with measures such as AZT and trimethoprim-sulfamethoxazole has which of the following direct effects on AIDS in the adult population?
  **A.** Decreased incidence of AIDS
  **B.** Increased incidence of AIDS
  **C.** Decreased prevalence of AIDS
  **D.** Increased prevalence of AIDS
  **E.** No effect on incidence or prevalence of AIDS

**47.** An increase in prevalence of a disease may be related to which of the following?
  **A.** Decreased incidence
  **B.** Shortened duration
  **C.** Increased mortality
  **D.** Decreased cure
  **E.** None of the above

**48.** Town B has a higher crude mortality proportion as a result of lung cancer in men than town A. However, the sex-specific, age-standardized mortality from lung cancer is higher in town A than town B. What conclusion may be drawn from these data?
  **A.** There were more deaths from lung cancer in town A than town B
  **B.** There were more deaths from lung cancer in town B than town A
  **C.** Town A has a younger age distribution than town B

**D.** Town B has a younger age distribution than town A

**E.** None of the above conclusions may be made with certainty from the data given

**49.** In use of the epidemiologic method of investigation, which of the following is done first?
**A.** Deduce the causative agent of the disease under study
**B.** Determine the population at risk of the disease under study
**C.** Formulate a case definition for the disease under study
**D.** Tabulate cases of the disease under study
**E.** Orient cases of the disease under study to time, place, and person

**50.** The national notifiable disease surveillance system is most useful for which of the following purposes?
**A.** Describing long-term trends of a disease
**B.** Detecting all cases of a disease in a geographic region
**C.** Rapidly detecting disease in an outbreak
**D.** Representative detection of disease
**E.** None of the above

**51.** Hypothesis testing regarding a possible causal association is generally limited to which of the following study types?
**A.** Review of case reports
**B.** Ecologic study
**C.** Cross-sectional study
**D.** Case–control study
**E.** None of the above

**52.** Which of the following factors is **LEAST** important for the success of a screening program?
**A.** The prevalence of the detectable preclinical phase of the disease in the screened population
**B.** The sensitivity of the screening test
**C.** The specificity of the screening test
**D.** Acceptance of the screening procedure by the screened population
**E.** How closely the characteristics of the screened population represent the general population

**53.** Proportion of motor vehicle accidents in 1985 by drivers' age:

| Driver's Age | **Proportion of All Motor Vehicle Accidents in 1985 by Age Category (%)** |
|---|---|
| 15–19 | 29.7 |
| 20–29 | 28.9 |
| 30–39 | 11.4 |
| 40–49 | 11.9 |
| 50–59 | 8.3 |
| 60 + | 9.8 |

The inference drawn from this information is that **the greatest *risk* of accidents occurs in drivers 15 to 19 years old.** Indicate which of the following choices best describes this inference. Please justify your answer using only the data presented in the table above.
A. The inference is correct
B. The inference is incorrect because it is *not* based on incidence
C. The inference is incorrect because it does *not* evaluate statistical significance
D. The inference is incorrect because of self-selection of study participants
E. The inference is incorrect because it fails to include data on alcohol consumption

**54.** The capacity of a test or procedure to screen as "negative" those **NOT** having a specific disease is
A. validity
B. sensitivity
C. specificity
D. positive predictive value
E. negative predictive value

**55.** California Highway Patrol statistics reveal that drivers of sports cars are involved in more accidents per mile driven when compared to drivers of sedans. The inference that Nellie Godiva, who drives a red Corvette, is at higher risk of being involved in a traffic accident when compared to Normal Elder, who drives a silver Oldsmobile Cutlass, is
A. correct
B. incorrect, because population data *cannot* be used to make predictions for individuals

**C.** incorrect, because the difference in horsepower for the two cars is **NOT** statistically significant

**D.** incorrect, because Norman's blood alcohol is usually around 0.25%

**E.** incorrect, because Nellie drives Norman crazy

**56.** Glaucoma is a progressive eye disease that causes blindness if not treated early. In a glaucoma detection program, two interpretations of screening data were considered. Both used the same subjects and data. Interpretation A used a cutoff that produced a larger number of *false positive* test results than interpretation B. Select the most correct answer regarding the test validity expected using each of the interpretations.

**A.** The sensitivity provided using interpretation A is greater than that for B

**B.** The specificity provided by interpretation A is greater than that for B

**C.** The sensitivity and specificity for both interpretations will be identical

**D.** The sensitivity plus the specificity must equal 1.00 using both interpretations

**E.** The sensitivity and specificity *cannot* be compared using the data provided

**57.** Select the most correct statement regarding the meaning of a statistically significant result obtained in a case–control study.

**A.** The result was explained by systematic error

**B.** The result *cannot* be explained by random error

**C.** The null hypothesis *cannot* be true

**D.** The result was produced by a biologic effect

**E.** None of the answers are correct

**58.** Select the method that is **NOT** useful for controlling (removing the effects of) confounding factors in case–control studies.

**A.** Selecting a study population having a homogeneous range of the confounding factor

**B.** Randomized assignment of exposure

**C.** Standardization regarding the confounding factor

**D.** Use of multivariable (multivariate) analysis methods

**E.** Stratification of comparison groups into narrow ranges of the confounding factor

**59.** In a *case–control* study of ovarian cancer and past diet, cases and controls were matched for age, reproductive history, and social class. The results of the study indicate that cases and controls differed significantly regarding past animal fat intake, use of birth control pills, and use of alcohol. Which of the following **CANNOT** be cited as a factor that would account for the differences observed?
 **A.** Gender (sex)
 **B.** Age
 **C.** Reproductive history
 **D.** Social class
 **E.** A through D

**60.** The ecologic fallacy is which of the following?
 **A.** The assumption that an exposure measured at the same time as an outcome was the cause of the outcome
 **B.** The assumption that variables associated on an aggregate level also are associated on an individual level
 **C.** The assumption that environmental factors are responsible for the majority of human disease
 **D.** The error that occurs when environmental exposure is measured in systematically different ways for the study groups
 **E.** The error that occurs when comparison groups differ in a systematic way that influences the outcome of investigation

**61.** Observational cohort studies have which of the following advantages over other studies?
 **A.** Require relatively few study subjects
 **B.** Obtain results relatively quickly
 **C.** Allow study of more than one effect of an exposure
 **D.** Are able to ascertain the effects of a treatment for the disease studied
 **E.** Are optimal for study of rare diseases with long latency

**62.** The two **MOST** important values usually necessary as a description of the frequency distribution of a series of observations are
 **A.** standard deviation and mean
 **B.** median and variance
 **C.** mode and range
 **D.** range and mean
 **E.** size of sample and standard deviation

**63.** For measurements that follow a normal distribution, the values that will differ from the mean by more than three times the standard deviation are approximately

   **A.** 1 in 10
   **B.** 1 in 25
   **C.** 1 in 55
   **D.** 1 in 100
   **E.** 1 in 370

**64.** Assuming a normal curve, the proportion of observations that lie within three times the standard deviation from the mean is

   **A.** 99.73%
   **B.** 95.45%
   **C.** 12.20%
   **D.** 68.27%
   **E.** 00.27%

**Questions 65–68:**
A group of 215 children are found to have hemoglobin values ranging from 9.0 to 14.9 g/100 mL, with a mean of 11.94 g/100 mL. The distribution is relatively normal with a standard deviation of 1.0 g/100 mL. On the basis of this study, one can conclude that

**65.** The average hemoglobin value for the group is

   **A.** 9.94 g/100 mL
   **B.** 10.94 g/100 mL
   **C.** 11.94 g/100 mL
   **D.** 12.93 g/100 mL
   **E.** 13.94 g/100 mL

**66.** The percentage of hemoglobin values larger than the average for the group is

   **A.** 20%
   **B.** 30%
   **C.** 40%
   **D.** 50%
   **E.** 60%

**67.** The percentage of hemoglobin values lying between plus one standard deviation and minus one standard deviation is
 **A.** 15%
 **B.** 25%
 **C.** 33⅓%
 **D.** 68%
 **E.** 75%

**68.** The percentage of hemoglobin values that is below minus 2 standard deviations from the mean is
 **A.** 1%
 **B.** 2%
 **C.** 4%
 **D.** 8%
 **E.** 16%

**69.** Advantages of retrospective studies include all of the following **EXCEPT**
 **A.** rather inexpensive to carry out
 **B.** number of subjects can often be rather small
 **C.** results can be obtained rather quickly
 **D.** yields rates rather than ratios
 **E.** frequently identify more than one risk

**Questions 70–74:**
For each of the following five numbered statements, select the ONE lettered heading that is most closely associated with it. Each lettered heading may be selected once, more than once, or not at all.

 **A.** Incidence rate
 **B.** Point prevalence rate
 **C.** Period prevalence rate
 **D.** Proportional mortality rate
 **E.** Neonatal mortality rate

**70.** Death under 28 days of age divided by live births

**71.** Deaths assigned to a specific disease, divided by all deaths

**72.** New cases of a disease diagnosed during a given period, divided by midperiod population

**73.** Existing cases of disease at a single moment in time divided by population at the same moment

**74.** Current cases, new and old, of a disease occurring during a given interval of the month, divided by the midinterval population

# Public Health Methods

## Answers and Discussion

1. **(B)** Motor vehicle accidents are a leading cause of death for children aged 2 years and above. Most such fatalities are preventable by use of child restraints in automobiles. Counseling parents regarding use of a car seat, and safety belts for older children, is an important preventive measure. (**Ref. 1,** pp. xxxix–xlv)

2. **(C)** A serum total cholesterol is indicated every 5 years, starting by the age of 35 years, or earlier. The other preventive measures listed are recommended by some major authorities, starting after the age of 50 years, except for urinalysis, which is recommended to start after the age of 60 years. (**Ref. 4,** p. 163)

3. **(C)** For a slender white woman who is postmenopausal, there is an increased risk of osteoporosis. It is thus appropriate to discuss estrogen replacement therapy with her and ask about possible contraindications (eg, history of breast cancer or active liver disease). Another important measure for her would be discussion of an exercise program. The other measures listed could be helpful for certain specific individuals but may not be needed in her case. (**Ref. 1,** pp. 239–242)

4. **(B)** Treatment of a disease that is already present to reduce the severity of its consequences is secondary prevention. Antiviral therapy for AIDS is direct treatment of the disease and thus is secondary prevention. Tertiary prevention would be limitation of disability through rehabilitation. (**Ref. 3,** pp. 56–57, **Ref. 2,** pp. 4–5, 119)

**5. (A)** Treatment that prevents development of a disease is primary prevention. Treating a person with AIDS using trimethoprim-sulfamethoxazole is intended to prevent *Pneumocystis carinii* pneumonia. Thus, it is a primary preventive measure for pneumonia and a secondary prevention for AIDS. (**Ref. 3,** pp. 56–57, **Ref. 2,** pp. 4–5)

**6. (B)** Successful secondary prevention measures generally have no direct effect on disease incidence. Instead, secondary prevention can alter prevalence by changing the duration of disease. Secondary prevention measures for otherwise fatal diseases can increase prevalence by increasing duration when treatment prevents death but does not offer a cure. (**Ref. 3,** pp. 56–57)

**7. (C)** Incidence measures risk of a disease within a defined population and time period. The terms risk and cumulative incidence are frequently used synonymously in the health literature. (**Ref. 3,** pp. 22–23)

**8. (E); 9. (B); 10. (C)** The annual prevalence of X is computed using the number of existing cases of disease during 1993 (old and new cases = 1100) as the numerator and the entire population at the beginning of the year as the denominator. The risk of disease X is the annual incidence of disease X during 1993 and is equal to the number of new cases of disease X (100) divided by the population at risk at the beginning of the year (100,000 minus the 1000 existing cases), so it is 100 divided by 99,000, or 101. Risk of death, or mortality proportion, is deaths from a specific cause divided by the population at risk of death from that cause at the beginning of the time period. (**Ref. 3,** pp. 22, 42, 43, 51)

**11. (D); 12. (C); 13. (A); 14. (B)** Viability is the capacity of an agent to survive in a defined environment outside the host. Virulence is the propensity of an agent to produce severe and fatal disease. Pathogenicity is the property of an agent that determines the extent to which overt disease is produced in an infected population, ie, the capacity of an agent to produce the functional, morphologic, and pathologic changes that cause symptomatic disease. Infectivity is the agent characteristic that embodies capability to enter, survive, and multiply in the host. (**Ref. 3,** p. 89)

**15. (A)** A fomite is an article that conveys infection to others because it has been contaminated by pathogenic organisms. Examples include handkerchieves, drinking glasses, door handles, clothing, and toys. **(Ref. 3,** p. 89)

**16. (C); 17. (D); 18. (A); 19. (B)** Ecologic studies use groups as the unit of comparison, rather than individuals, when assessing relationships between two or more characteristics (eg, cancer and sale of beef). The "ecologic fallacy" occurs when bias is introduced by assuming that an inference that is observed at the group level also applies to the individual. Cross-sectional studies simultaneously evaluate exposure and outcome in a population. Observational studies can be categorized as cohort or case–control. In a case–control study, the risk of exposure to a cause by those with a health problem (cases) is compared with the risk of exposure of those who do not have the health problem (controls). It is a retrospective study when outcomes that are rare or have a long latency or incubation period are identified and compared with controls. Cohort studies begin with a case group made up of individuals exposed to the hypothesized cause of a health problem. The comparison group is one that is not exposed but has similar demographic, behavioral, and biologic characteristics. The groups are compared and characterized according to the rates at which the health problem occurs in each group. **(Ref. 2,** pp. 24–25)

**20. (C)** Specificity is the probability that a person not having a disease will test negative on a screening test for that disease. **(Ref. 3,** p. 238)

**21. (A)** The crude birth rate (CBR) uses all births as the numerator and the total population, regardless of gender or age, as the denominator. The general fertility rate (GFR) also uses all births as the numerator but is based on a denominator comprising all women of childbearing age, most often defined as women 15 to 44 years of age. The age-specific fertility rate (ASFR) is calculated using births to women in a specific age interval as the numerator and women in the same age interval as the denominator. The total fertility rate (TFR) is the sum of all the age-specific fertility rates by single years of age. **(Ref. 2,** p. 43)

**22. (C)** Fertility, in its most specific sense, refers to the actual birth of living offspring. Fecundity is the capacity to bear children, and fecundability is the probability of conceiving in a given month. (**Ref. 2,** p. 44)

**23. (C)** Life expectancy in the world is generally increasing. In recent years, Japan has become the country with the highest life expectancy at birth for males, reaching 73.8 years in 1981 and 75.5 years in 1986, among 40 nations for which current information is available. (**Ref. 2,** p. 48)

**24. (B)** The movement of people to cities (urbanization) is one of the dominant characteristics of population change of the 20th century. At the beginning of the century, fewer than one out of every seven persons in the world lived in a city. As we near the year 2000, more than 40% of the world's population is found in urban areas. (**Ref. 2,** p. 51)

**25. (B)** With birth rates having apparently held steady during most of human history, we must look to decreases in death rates to explain why growth rates have shot up the last 200 years. The change is mainly due to improvements in public sanitation, advances in agriculture, and the control of infectious diseases, which have resulted in a decline in death rates, particularly in infant and child mortality. (**Ref. 5,** p. 65)

**26. (A)** The high percentage of people under 15 is indicative of the explosive growth potential of most developing nations. In most developing nations this percentage is 40% to 50%. By contrast, the percentage of people under 15 in most industrialized countries is 16% to 25%. (**Ref. 5,** p. 71)

**27. (B)** Since birth rates represent additions to a population and death rates represent subtractions, a change in population size is represented by the difference between the two, ie, by the growth rate of that population. Growth rates can be calculated quite simply by subtracting the death rate from the birth rate and are normally expressed as a percent, not per 1000 as in birth and death rates. (**Ref. 5,** p. 60)

**28. (C)** One of the more newly identified hantaviruses has been implicated as the cause of a new disease, hantavirus pulmonary syndrome (HPS), characterized by a prodrome of fever followed by rapidly developing noncardiac pulmonary edema and shock. Other hantaviruses had previously been associated with hemorrhagic fever with a renal syndrome. There have been instances of hantaviral transmission in laboratories housing and studying the rodent hosts. It is possible that there could be transmission from rodent bites or rodent contact with broken skin. However, the main mode of transmission in the United States has been from inhalation of aerosolized virus from rodent saliva, urine, or other excreta. **(Ref. 6)**

**29. (C)** *Cryptosporidium parvum,* a protozoan virtually unknown until 1976, first became widely known as a pathogen in AIDS patients. It has more recently caused outbreaks of gastrointestinal illness spread by swimming pools or drinking water in several communities. The amount of chlorine needed to kill *Cryptosporidium* oocytes is 640 times that necessary to kill *Giardia* cysts. It is not feasible to maintain such high levels of chlorine in the water when so few are at risk for more serious infections. The portal of entry is thought to be oral. Use of barrier protection when having sexual relations with a *Cryptosporidium*-infected person, particularly with anal contact, is advised. Strict hand washing can break the fecal-oral transmission route. **(Ref. 7)**

**30. (C)** For a screening test to be effective, the most important single factor to consider is that it have a high predictive value positive. This will be related to both the sensitivity and the specificity of the test and also to the incidence of the disease in the population being tested. If a disease is very rare in the screened population, the predictive value of a positive test may be low, even with both very high sensitivity and specificity. Thus, part of a surveillance system can entail selection of populations at higher risk and targeting them for screening. Some other important attributes for an effective surveillance program are simplicity, acceptability, and flexibility. **(Ref. 2,** pp. 16, 17)

**31. (B)** Calculation of incidence of disease requires knowledge of the number of cases occurring in a specific population (the numerator) and the size of that population (the denominator). Data from a population-based registry for a geographic region will allow calculation of incidence for that region. The registry will give the number of cases, and the size of the population will be available from census data. Neither hospital records nor a disease case registry have a well-defined population from which the cases are derived. Thus, they cannot be used to find incidence, as the denominator information is not available. Mortality records do not show cases that are still alive and do not have the proper numerator information. (**Ref. 11,** pp. 29–32)

32. **(A)** Active surveillance may find cases of disease that would otherwise have been missed. Thus, it increases sensitivity. On the other hand, cases found may not be quite as representative of the population at large. Also, clinicians may report potential cases prior to verification, and some of these people may subsequently turn out not to have the disease. This can decrease the specificity and the predictive value positive. However, this decrease may be acceptable in an epidemic situation, when early detection of the disease is most important. (**Ref. 2,** pp. 16, 17)

33. **(D)** When an outbreak is being investigated, disease control and preventive measures should have priority over investigative steps. Measures to control a potential health problem may need to be implemented while other investigative results are being waited for (eg, by isolating individuals with a potentially infectious disease). However, there are generally some grounds on which to base decisions (eg, using clinical signs and symptoms to make a presumptive diagnosis while awaiting culture results).

The subsequent investigation should include specific steps. Initially a case definition needs to be formulated and the diagnosis confirmed for cases. This will allow investigators to verify the existence of an epidemic by making comparisons with data on the prior endemic level of disease. Description of the population characteristics of time, place, and persons affected by disease will be important. Further steps include formulation and testing of hypothesis and searching for additional cases of the disease. Again, the ultimate purpose of the investigation is disease control and prevention, and these should have priority over the investigative steps. (**Ref. 2,** pp. 22–24)

34. **(E)** This is a case–control study that does not include the size of the populations at risk. Therefore, incidence cannot be calculated. The measure that would be useful here would be the odds ratio (which is $[647 \times 27]/[2 \times 622]$). The odds ratio is an approxima-

tion of the relative risk, which may be obtained in cohort studies. The relative risk is the ratio of the incidence in the exposed cohort to the incidence in the unexposed cohort. Calculation of incidence requires knowledge of both the number of cases occurring in a specific population for the numerator and the size of that population for the denominator. The case–control study does not have population size. (**Ref. 2**, pp. 27–29; **Ref. 11**, pp. 23–32, 36–38, 62–64)

**35. (B)** Case–control studies are especially useful in studying rare diseases. In a cohort study, rare diseases could require very large cohorts to be certain of finding a significant number of cases of the disease. On the other hand, a cohort study can be useful to evaluate multiple effects from a single exposure. The case–control study is not able to evaluate the mechanism of disease. To study the effects of treatment for a disease, an interventional study is required. In such studies, different cohorts receive the treatment and others placebo (or other standard treatment, for comparison). (**Ref. 12**, pp. 20–22; **Ref. 11**, pp. 51–69)

**36. (B)** The relative risk is the ratio of the incidence in those exposed to the incidence in the unexposed. If the following table is used:

**Disease**

|  |  | Present | Absent |
|---|---|---|---|
| **Known exposure** | Present | a | b |
|  | Absent | c | d |

the relative risk will be [a/(a+b)] divided by [c/(c+d)]. It should be noted that the odds ratio can provide an unbiased estimate of the relative risk when the disease is uncommon, as seen here. The odds ratio is computed using the formula a·d/b·c (answer **A**). (**Ref. 2**, pp. 28, 29)

**37. (B)** The ELISA test is repeated because of the high number of false positives (ie, low specificity). Repeating the test greatly increases the predictive value positive. However, there is a slight chance that the test may be falsely negative, and this chance is increased by the serial testing. Thus, it slightly decreases the sensitivity. The initial screening by ELISA is very sensitive, but not so specific. The subsequent tests are both very sensitive and very specific. They are performed later because they are more expensive. Cost is controlled by screening using the ELISA test. (**Ref. 8,** pp. 58–66)

38. **(C)** The incidence rate is expressed as cases over person-time. The numerator is cases in a population with onset during a specific time period. The denominator is the sum of the time periods of observation for all the individuals in the population. This denominator can be approximated by the product of the population size and the average time period of observation for individuals in the population. However, the observation period for individuals may vary. In particular, when the first occurrence of a disease is being measured, the observation period ends with onset of disease. Thus, use of the sum of time periods of observation for all the individuals is most accurate.

   Note that cumulative incidence is often mislabeled as an incidence rate. Cumulative incidence is answer **A**, cases in a population with onset during a specific time period, divided by the population size at the start of the time period. Cumulative incidence is dimensionless, while the true incidence rate has units of reciprocal time. Also, note that incidence looks specifically at the cases with onset in the specific time period and not at cases that existed before. This is as opposed to prevalence, which is a measurement of the proportion of people with disease at a specific time. (**Ref. 11,** pp. 23–32)

39. **(A)** The "infant mortality rate" is not a true rate because infant deaths in a year are not necessarily from the population of live births for that year. An infant death is any death prior to the first birthday. Many infant deaths may be among infants born the preceding year. A true rate may be represented as a numerator composed of cases measured in a time interval over a denominator that may be represented as the product of the size of the population from which the cases were drawn and the average time interval during which the individuals were susceptible to the disease. The denominator is also the sum of the time periods of observation for all the individuals in the population. For a true rate, the cases in the numerator must be drawn from the population in the denominator. In addition, a proportion is represented as cases drawn from a population with onset in a time interval over the size of the population from which the cases were drawn. (**Ref. 11,** pp. 23–29)

**40. (E)** A hazards rate is essentially an incidence rate calculated using the shortest possible time interval. In practice, this may realistically be a day, a week, or even a year. The hazards rate is used when the incidence of disease (or risk of disease) is changing with time. This is particularly likely during an outbreak, or epidemic. (**Ref. 9,** pp. 243, 246)

**41. (D)** The ratio of the cumulative incidence proportion for an exposed population to that of an unexposed population is the relative risk. When the incidence rate or hazards rate is nearly constant, the incidence rate ratio and hazards rate ratio will be approximately equal to the relative risk. The odds ratio is approximately equal to the relative risk when the disease is rare. On the other hand, a risk difference is found by subtracting the cumulative incidence proportion for an unexposed population from that of an exposed population. While it is determined by the same values as the relative risk, the risk difference is a risk in its own right and can never be equal to the relative risk. (**Ref. 11,** pp. 36–38, 63, 64; **Ref. 9,** pp. 246, 252, 253)

**42. (B)** The disease-specific case-fatality proportion is given by deaths from the specific disease divided by the total number of cases of the specified disease. This gives a measure of risk of death from the disease among those with the disease. Note that it is sometimes called a case-fatality rate, though it is actually a proportion. Use of the disease-specific case-fatality proportion to represent risk of death among those with the disease is most accurate if there is a short period of increased risk after onset of the disease. If there is a long period of increased risk, use of the mortality rate among those with the illness will be preferable, since this will allow the actual time at risk for each individual to be taken into account. The disease-specific mortality proportion is represented by deaths from the disease over the population at risk of death. Thus, it is the risk of death from the disease in the general population. The disease-specific proportion of mortality is shown by deaths from a specific cause over deaths from all causes. It is not a risk measure. (**Ref. 11,** pp. 23–32, 72–74)

**43. (B)** Risk of dying from a specific disease in a general population is measured with the disease-specific mortality proportion. This is the number of deaths resulting from the specific disease divided by the size of the entire population at risk of death. Two of the other measures have the same numerator but different denominators. One of these is the disease-specific proportion of mortality, with the denominator being all deaths in the population. The other is the disease-specific case-fatality proportion, with the denominator being all cases of the specific disease. (**Ref. 10, pp.** 71–75)

**44.** (**E**)  Risk of developing a disease is **BEST** measured using the cumulative incidence of the disease in the population. Here risk is considered to be the probability of an individual's developing the disease in a specified time interval. This evaluates risk only on the basis of belonging to the population under study and does not consider subpopulations with increased likelihood of exposure to AIDS. For instance, risk among homosexual men would **BEST** be assessed by measuring the incidence in this subpopulation, if the subpopulation size were known. One problem is that the size of this subpopulation may not be known, making such a risk assessment more difficult. (**Ref. 10,** p. 138)

**45.** (**C**)  Proportional mortality studies do not measure risk of dying, since the denominator is deaths from all causes rather than the living population. The findings given merely show that a larger proportion of deaths in Uganda may be attributed to causes other than cancer. This could be due to either a protective effect against dying from cancer or an increased risk of dying from some other cause. The data given do not allow differentiation between these possibilities. There is also no data on the prevalence of cancer or the cancer-specific mortality rate. (**Ref. 11,** pp. 72–74)

**46.** (**D**)  When a chronic, incurable disease that may be fatal is so treated that life is lengthened, the net effect from treatment alone is an increase in the prevalence of AIDS, above what it otherwise would be. Thus, an increase in prevalence may not be a bad thing when it is due to longer survival, as it is here. Incidence will not be affected among adults, although it may go down as a result of less maternal transmission to infants. To decrease the incidence of disease, and subsequently the prevalence, measures to prevent AIDS would be needed. (**Ref. 9,** pp. 27–29)

**47.** (**D**)  Increased prevalence of a disease may be related to a decrease in curing the disease. It is directly related to incidence and duration of the disease so increases when these increase. On the other hand, it is negatively related to things that lead an individual with disease to no longer have the disease, including both a cure or mortality. (**Ref. 9,** pp. 27–29)

**48.** **(C)** Lung cancer is more likely to cause mortality in older persons. Age standardization gives a relative increase in the mortality proportion for town A compared with town B. This must be due to town A's having a younger age distribution than town B. The actual number of deaths resulting from lung cancer depends on the population sizes of towns A and B, and one cannot be certain what these are just from the data given. (**Ref. 11,** pp. 41–44; **Ref. 9,** pp. 32–34)

**49.** **(C)** Epidemiologic reasoning follows a specific sequence. First the epidemiologist must specifically define what will be considered a case of the disease to be studied. Next cases are counted and oriented to time, place, and person. Then the population at risk of the disease is determined, and rates of incidence are calculated. Finally inferences are drawn regarding matters such as the causative agent of the disease and factors in the host or environment that influence risk of the disease. (**Ref. 2,** pp. 22–24)

**50.** **(A)** The national notifiable disease surveillance system is particularly useful for describing seasonal and long-term trends of disease. It is simple, acceptable, and flexible. However, it is not as sensitive as efforts by a local health agency can be. It is also not as timely or representative. (**Ref. 2,** p. 16)

**51.** **(D)** Testing of a hypothesis may be done using observational studies such as a case–control study or a cohort study. The other options given, such as ecologic studies and cross-sectional studies, are sometimes referred to as hypothesis-generating studies. As this term implies, such studies are useful for generating hypotheses about possible associations but not for testing such hypotheses. (**Ref. 11,** pp. 51–74; **Ref. 9,** pp. 37–46)

**52.** **(E)** To maximize success, the screened population should be at higher risk for the specified disease than the general population. Sensitivity, specificity, and the prevalence of the detectable preclinical phase (frequently measured as disease incidence) all contribute to the positive predictive value. (**Ref. 57**)

**53.** **(B)** Risk is the proportion of a population at risk that experiences an event (incidence). In this example, no data about the population at risk are provided, making a calculation of risk impossible. (**Ref. 14, p. 51**)

**54.** **(C)** Specificity is true negatives/(true negatives + false positives), or true negatives divided by all those without the disease. This is the proportion of subjects without disease who test negative, or the capacity of a test or procedure to screen as "negative" those *not* having a specific disease. (**Ref. 14, p. 220**)

**55.** **(B)** Use of population data to make predictions for individual members of groups can result in an invalid stereotype known as "ecologic fallacy." (**Ref. 70, p. 186**)

**56.** **(A)** The greater likelihood of false positive results for interpretation A is a consequence of the smaller probability of false negatives created by reducing the cut-point used to classify results as suspicious for glaucoma. Shifting the cut-point for the screening test can be used to trade sensitivity for specificity (and vice versa) by trading false positive and false negative test results. (**Ref. 14, p. 219**)

**57.** **(E)** A statistically significant result is one in which the probability of obtaining a finding showing a similar or greater difference from the null value is less than or equal to the stated alpha level (not likely the result of chance). Statistically significant results can and are produced by either random error that is uncommon, but possible; systematic error; or the effect (frequently biologic) that gave rise to the alternate hypothesis. (**Ref. 62, pp. 31–37**)

**58.** **(B)** Randomization is only possible in experimental studies and cannot be used in case–control studies. (**Ref. 11, p. 109**)

**59.** **(A)** Ovarian cancer is female-specific; therefore, measurement of an association between characteristics of cases and controls mandates use of female subjects only. Matching in case–control studies can be used to improve the efficiency (statistical power) of the investigation but will *not* eliminate confounding by the matched factor. In this example, matching on age, reproductive history, and social class would be expected to introduce or translate confounding, producing a systematic error that would likely bias toward the null hypothesis. Matching in case–control studies should be accompanied by a procedure in the analysis that eliminates the confounding produced or translated by the matching process. (**Ref. 11,** pp. 243, 244)

**60. (B)** The ecologic fallacy is the assumption that variables associated on an aggregate level also are associated on an individual level. Ecologic studies look at groups, such as populations of countries. They compare proportions of people who have certain exposures with proportions who have certain diseases in different groups (correlation may be used). While this comparison may suggest a possible association, it is not a certainty. There is no way to be certain that the people who have the exposure history are the same ones who develop the disease. (**Ref. 2,** p. 24)

**61. (C)** Cohort studies take one group with a known exposure and another comparable group without the exposure and follow the groups over time. A relatively large number of subjects are required and a relatively long time in comparison with a case–control study. Because of these factors, case–control studies are better for study of rare diseases with long latency. For evaluating a treatment, an interventional study rather than an observational cohort study would be needed. (**Ref. 11,** pp. 51–74; **Ref. 9,** pp. 37–46)

**62. (A)** The most important values in describing the frequency distribution of a series of observations are the mean and standard deviation. (**Ref. 13,** pp. 36–40)

**63. (E)** When considering a normal distribution, 99.73% of your observations will be within ± three standard deviations from the mean. Values more or less than this are very rare. (**Ref. 13,** p. 68)

**64. (A)** Plus or minus 3 SD contain 99.73%; plus or minus 2 SD contain 95.45%; plus or minus 1 SD contain 68.27%. (**Ref. 13,** p. 68)

**65. (C)** The "average" in statistical terms is known as the "mean." (**Ref. 13,** p. 38)

**66. (D)** With this large sample size, 50% will have values larger than the average. (**Ref. 13,** p. 71)

**67.** **(D)** A standard deviation of one above and below the mean contains 68% of the total sample size. Plus or minus two standard deviations contains approximately 95.5%, and plus or minus three standard deviations contains approximately 99.7% of the total sample size. **(Ref. 13, p. 71)**

**68.** **(B)** Approximately 2% of the sample is below minus two standard deviations from the mean. **(Ref. 13, p. 71)**

**69.** **(D)** In fact, a disadvantage to retrospective studies is that they cannot yield rates, only ratios (that is, relative risk). Other disadvantages are the bias of recall and the problem of selecting control groups. It is true, however, that retrospective studies are relatively inexpensive, relatively rapid, and consequently can be easily repeated. **(Ref. 14, pp. 163, 169)**

**70.** **(E)** Neonatal mortality rate is death under 28 days of age divided by live births. In each definition the denominator is the population at risk. The only way to get into the numerator is by acquiring the condition. **(Ref. 15, pp. 56, 57)**

**71.** **(D)** The proportional mortality rate is defined as each death assigned to a specific disease divided by all deaths. **(Ref. 15, pp. 56, 57)**

**72.** **(A)** Incidence rate is based on new events (ie, new cases of a disease diagnosed during a given period). **(Ref. 15, pp. 56, 57)**

**73.** **(B)** Point prevalence rate is based on cases of a disease existing in a theoretical moment of time. **(Ref. 15, pp. 56, 57)**

**74.** **(C)** Period prevalence rate is based on current cases, new and old, occurring in a given time interval. **(Ref. 15, pp. 56, 57)**

# 2

# Communicable Diseases

75. A 33-year-old white man traveled to South America for 3 days. Within hours of his return he had onset of watery diarrhea and abdominal cramping. What is the most likely etiology?
    A. *Yersinia*
    B. *Escherichia coli*
    C. *Giardia*
    D. *Salmonella*
    E. *Entamoeba*

76. Prophylaxis of traveler's diarrhea can best be accomplished by
    A. trimethoprim-sulfamethoxazole
    B. penicillin
    C. metronidazole
    D. iodochlorhydroxyquin (Entero-Vioform)
    E. amphotericin-B

77. Effective preventive measures for traveler's diarrhea include all of the following **EXCEPT**
    A. avoidance of ice-chilled beverages
    B. avoidance of raw vegetables
    C. use of water treated with two to four drops of 5% chlorine bleach per quart of water

    **D.** use of water treated with five to ten drops of 2% tincture of iodine per quart of water

    **E.** purifying water through a ceramic filter

**78.** Which of the following vaccines may be required for travel in endemic areas?

    **A.** Yellow fever vaccine

    **B.** Smallpox vaccine

    **C.** Meningococcal vaccine

    **D.** Japanese encephalitis vaccine

    **E.** Typhoid fever

**79.** Which of the following is **NOT** a manifestation associated with various *Escherichia coli* organisms?

    **A.** Hemorrhagic colitis

    **B.** Hemolytic uremic syndrome

    **C.** Meningitis

    **D.** Watery diarrhea

    **E.** Fever

**80.** Which of the following vaccines for nonimmune travelers is recommended for pregnant women?

    **A.** Measles, mumps, rubella vaccine

    **B.** Yellow fever vaccine

    **C.** Oral typhoid vaccine

    **D.** Tetanus toxoid vaccine

    **E.** Polio vaccine

**81.** In general, for nonimmune travelers who are HIV (human immunodeficiency virus)-positive, the following vaccinations are contraindicated **EXCEPT** which one?

    **A.** Oral polio vaccine

    **B.** Measles, mumps, rubella vaccine

    **C.** Oral typhoid vaccine

    **D.** Yellow fever vaccine

    **E.** BCG vaccine

**82.** For immunizations in a healthy infant whose immunization schedule is up to date, all of the following vaccines may be appropriate for the 6-month visit in nonepidemic years **EXCEPT**
   **A.** oral polio vaccine
   **B.** diphtheria, pertussis, tetanus vaccine
   **C.** measles, mumps, rubella vaccine
   **D.** *Haemophilus influenzae,* type B vaccine
   **E.** hepatitis B

**83.** The oral typhoid vaccine would be most appropriate for travelers in which of the following situations?
   **A.** Children under the age of 2 years
   **B.** Travelers on brief stops in endemic areas
   **C.** Women in the first trimester of pregnancy
   **D.** HIV-positive travelers
   **E.** Elderly travelers to Europe

**84.** Immune globulin should be withheld or given with caution in all of the following situations **EXCEPT**
   **A.** in persons with sensitivity to mercury
   **B.** in persons receiving MMR concurrently
   **C.** in persons with severe thrombocytopenia
   **D.** in persons receiving OPV concurrently
   **E.** in persons with an allergy to thimerosal

**85.** Which is the most appropriate situation for the administration of measles (rubeola) immunization?
   **A.** Travelers with HIV infection visiting an endemic area
   **B.** Americans born before 1957
   **C.** Pregnant women in endemic areas
   **D.** Persons with congenital immunodeficiency
   **E.** A 9-month-old infant in a nonendemic area

**86.** A 21-year-old college student presented to student health services with complaints of cough and fever for a few days. On physical examination, an erythematous maculopapular rash was seen, and Koplik's spots were present on the oral mucosa. Which of the following is true concerning this illness?
   **A.** This illness is more common and more severe in children, compared with infants or adults

**B.** In the typical form, the rash appears first on the torso and then spreads to the extremities

**C.** Conjunctivitis, excessive lacrimation, and photophobia are common symptoms

**D.** Prompt administration of immune globulin soon after exposure does *not* alter the course of the illness

**E.** Antibody protection after infection lasts for only 2 to 3 years

**87.** The single most useful method to control measles (rubeola) in the United States has been
   **A.** isolation of exposed individuals
   **B.** good sanitation in crowded institutions
   **C.** enactment and enforcement of school immunization laws
   **D.** maintaining high levels of passive immunity
   **E.** controlling immunization status of travelers

**88.** Which of the following is true about current vaccinations for influenza?
   **A.** The World Health Organization makes recommendations every 4 to 5 years to the Centers for Disease Control and Prevention and vaccine manufacturers on the formulation of the vaccines
   **B.** An increased incidence of Guillain-Barré syndrome has been observed in association with the influenza vaccine in the past 10 years
   **C.** The most common current vaccines are trivalent, with two A strains and one B strain
   **D.** Vaccination of high-risk groups has only a modest effect on their mortality rates
   **E.** Young college-age adults living in apartments should be immunized

**89.** Control of influenza mortality in the United States has best been approached by
   **A.** isolation
   **B.** prophylaxis
   **C.** immunization of high-risk groups
   **D.** ultraviolet irradiation
   **E.** immunization of travelers to endemic areas

**90.** Which of the following is the **LEAST** likely mode of transmission for varicella?
A. Airborne droplets
B. Direct contact
C. Fomites
D. Blood exposure
E. School contacts

**91.** Which of the following is **NOT** true about the prevention and treatment of *Haemophilis influenzae* infection?
A. Chemoprophylaxis with isoniazid for household contacts under 6 years of age has been recommended for patients with influenza meningitis
B. For normal, healthy infants, immunization for *H. influenzae* begins at 2 months of age
C. A three-stage vaccination is available for primary immunization and a booster
D. Treatment for life-threatening illnesses from *H. influenzae* may include both chloramphenicol and ampicillin
E. Protection with the vaccine lasts 5 to 10 years or longer

**92.** Which of the following statements is true concerning the epidemiology of *Haemophilis influenzae* infection?
A. Of cases of *H. influenzae* meningitis, 95% occur in children over 5 years of age
B. The incidence in Alaskan natives is 10 times the national average
C. The incidence of *H. influenzae* infection is lowest in the spring and fall
D. The incidence of *H. influenzae* meningitis is higher in whites than in blacks
E. The incidence of *H. influenzae* has been gradually declining over the past several decades

**93.** Concerning the epidemiology of pneumococcus (*Streptococcus pneumoniae*), which of the following statements is **NOT** true?
A. This organism is the most common cause of community acquired bacterial pneumonia
B. This organism is responsible for most cases of otitis media
C. This organism is one of the three most common causes of bacterial meningitis

**D.** This organism has a low case fatality rate in cases of meningitis because of great susceptibility to penicillin
**E.** Vaccination is recommended for seniors

**Questions 94 and 95:**
After an occurrence of fever and malaise, a 23-year-old pregnant woman in her first trimester presents with a history of a nonspecific maculopapular rash that lasted 3 days; she also had cervical lymphadenopathy.

**94.** Her unborn child may be at increased risk for which of the following congenital cardiac abnormalities?
**A.** Tetralogy of Fallot
**B.** Atrial septal defect
**C.** Myocardial necrosis
**D.** Aortic stenosis
**E.** Arrhythmias

**95.** The infant is also at increased risk for developing which of the following endocrinopathies?
**A.** Diabetes insipidus
**B.** Precocious puberty
**C.** Gout
**D.** Gigantism
**E.** Hypothyroidism

**96.** Which of the following methods has been most effective in the control and prevention of pertussis in the United States?
**A.** Isolation
**B.** Conferment of passive immunity
**C.** Conferment of active immunity
**D.** Restricted fomite transmission
**E.** Immunizing travelers

**97.** The most common cause of mortality associated with varicella infection in the adult population is
**A.** sepsis
**B.** pneumonia
**C.** encephalitis
**D.** meningitis
**E.** enteritis

**98.** Immunizations that are **NOT** appropriate for the human immunodeficiency (HIV)-positive, nonimmune traveler include
- **A.** measles, mumps, rubella vaccine
- **B.** inactivated polio vaccine
- **C.** bacille Calmette-Guérin vaccine
- **D.** pneumococcal vaccine
- **E.** injectable typhoid vaccine

**99.** Of the following means for immunizing, which one would be most appropriate for the HIV-positive traveler to endemic areas?
- **A.** Oral polio vaccine
- **B.** Bacille Calmette-Guérin vaccine
- **C.** Yellow fever vaccine
- **D.** Immune globulin
- **E.** Oral typhoid vaccine

**100.** Which of the following is the only virus that has been isolated from breast milk following a mother's immunization?
- **A.** Yellow fever
- **B.** Rubella
- **C.** Hepatitis B
- **D.** Polio
- **E.** Influenza

**101.** Precautions for the administration of oral polio vaccine include avoidance of vaccination in the presence of which of the following conditions?
- **A.** An immunodeficient household contact
- **B.** Prematurity
- **C.** Diarrhea
- **D.** Breast feeding
- **E.** Low-grade fever

**102.** In general, which of the following should be considered a precaution when administering the diphtheria-tetanus-pertussis vaccine?
- **A.** Family history of convulsions
- **B.** Family history of sudden infant death syndrome
- **C.** Temperature of 105°F (40.5°C)
- **D.** Prematurity
- **E.** Diarrhea

**103.** Current strategies recommended by the Centers for Disease Control and Prevention for epidemiologic control and prevention of sexually transmitted diseases in the US population include all of the following **EXCEPT**

    **A.** barrier methods
    **B.** contact tracing
    **C.** universal screening programs
    **D.** disease reporting
    **E.** monogamous relationships

**104.** Syphilis remains an important sexually transmitted disease in the United States, despite declining after reaching a peak in the latter half of the 1980s, because of each of the following **EXCEPT**

    **A.** its association with HIV transmission
    **B.** its escalating rate among male homosexuals
    **C.** its preventability and curability
    **D.** its effect on perinatal mortality and morbidity
    **E.** its impact on fertility

**105.** The following trends are reflective of gonorrhea infection in the United States in the last decade **EXCEPT**

    **A.** increase in the incidence among white homosexual males
    **B.** increase in the incidence among African-American teenagers
    **C.** decrease in the incidence among the US population
    **D.** Decrease in the incidence among white Americans
    **E.** Increase in the incidence among inner-city adolescents

**106.** Since the emergence of clinically significant penicillinase-producing *Neisseria gonorrhoeae* (PPNG), as well as of other forms of resistance, antibiotic resistance has been associated with all of the following drugs **EXCEPT**

    **A.** tetracyclines
    **B.** aminoglycosides
    **C.** third-generation cephalosporins
    **D.** penicillins
    **E.** doxycycline

**Questions 107–109:**
Match with the most closely associated organism.

**A.** *Neisseria gonorrhoeae*
**B.** *Chlamydia trachomatis*

**107.** Cause of the most common sexually transmitted bacterial genital infection

**108.** Plasmid-mediated resistance has hampered progress in treatment of

**109.** Chromosomally mediated resistance has hampered progress in treatment of

**Questions 110 and 111:**
A 30-year-old man comes into a community clinic with complaints of several lesions at the base of his penis. He is sexually active and has never had anything like this before. He complains that he has had these painful lesions for about 7 days.

**110.** What is the most likely causative organism?
**A.** *Chlamydia trachomatis*
**B.** Herpes simplex virus, type 2 (HSV-2)
**C.** *Haemophilus ducreyi*
**D.** *Treponema pallidum*
**E.** *Neisseria gonorrhoeae*

**111.** What will most likely provide the definitive diagnosis for this acute infection?
**A.** Serologic assay
**B.** Viral isolation from tissue culture
**C.** Tzanck preparation
**D.** Darkfield examination of tissue
**E.** Routine bacterial culture

**112.** Which of the following neoplasms has been strongly correlated with HSV-2?
**A.** Anal carcinoma
**B.** Vulvar carcinoma
**C.** Cervical carcinoma

**D.** Vaginal carcinoma
**E.** Penile carcinoma

**113.** Which of the following is an associated syndrome of genital HSV-2?
**A.** Epididymitis
**B.** Aseptic meningitis
**C.** Penile carcinoma
**D.** Prostatitis
**E.** Vulvavaginitis

**114.** What is the most appropriate management of genital HSV-2?
**A.** Erythromycin
**B.** Acyclovir
**C.** Ceftriaxone
**D.** Tetracycline
**E.** Amoxicillin

**115.** Which of the following is most true concerning herpes simplex virus, type 2 (HSV-2) infection and genital lesions?
**A.** In patients with HSV-2 antibodies, the majority noticed symptoms associated with their initial HSV-2 infection
**B.** In 75% of cases of confirmed HSV-2 transmission, no lesions were present at the time of transmission
**C.** HSV-2 infection is *not* associated with increased HIV risk among homosexuals
**D.** HSV-2 infection ranks number 3 as a cause of genital ulcerations
**E.** Neonatal herpes rate is declining

**116.** Efforts to aid in the diagnosis and control of subclinical human papilloma virus (HPV) infection include detecting all of the following **EXCEPT**
**A.** koilocytes on cytologic smears
**B.** HPV viral cultures
**C.** immunochemical stains for HPV antigen
**D.** HPV nucleic acid sequences (by PCR)
**E.** morphologic changes on colposcopy

**117.** Which of the following is true regarding HPV and subclinical infection?
  **A.** HPV is not usually transmitted in the absence of lesions
  **B.** Cervical cancer can be a sequela of HPV infection despite the absence of HPV lesions
  **C.** Subclinical HPV penile infections are thought to be uncommon
  **D.** Most of the 57 types of HPV are associated with genital infections
  **E.** HPV types 16 and 18 are most commonly associated with subclinical infection

**118.** For the control of hepatitis B infection (HBV), which of the following groups would it be most important to vaccinate to control transmission?
  **A.** Homosexual men
  **B.** Hemodialysis patients
  **C.** Institutionalized patients
  **D.** Health care workers
  **E.** Food handlers

**119.** The long-term effects of HBV infection include an increased risk for all of the following **EXCEPT**
  **A.** fulminant hepatitis
  **B.** cirrhosis
  **C.** chronic active hepatitis
  **D.** hepatocellular carcinoma
  **E.** hepatic thrombosis

**120.** A pregnant 23-year-old woman comes into a primary care clinic and receives a diagnosis of pelvic inflammatory disease. She is at **LEAST** risk for developing which of the following complications?
  **A.** Premature rupture of membranes
  **B.** Spontaneous abortion
  **C.** Chorioamnionitis
  **D.** Prematurity
  **E.** Low birth weight infant

**121.** To use available resources most effectively to prevent neonatal infection with herpes simplex virus (HSV), which of the following would be the best strategy?
  **A.** Cesarean delivery
  **B.** Screening prior to delivery for maternal HSV

    **C.** Reducing the duration of infectivity (decreasing viral transmission)

    **D.** Education regarding sexual practices of high-risk core groups

    **E.** Contact tracing

**122.** Human papilloma virus (HPV) infection has been strongly associated with all of the following neoplasms **EXCEPT**

    **A.** vulvar

    **B.** testicular

    **C.** anal

    **D.** cervical

    **E.** vaginal

**Questions 123–126:**

Match the cancer type with the most strongly associated infectious agent.

    **A.** human papilloma virus

    **B.** hepatitis B infection

    **C.** human immunodeficiency virus (HIV)

**123.** Penile carcinoma

**124.** Hepatocellular carcinoma

**125.** Non-Hodgkin's lymphoma

**126.** Anal carcinoma

**Questions 127 and 128:**

A 21-year-old man with signs of urethritis, conjunctivitis, and arthritis has just received a presumptive diagnosis of an accompanying sexually transmitted disease (STD).

**127.** What is the most likely organism to cause the associated STD?

    **A.** *Neisseria gonorrhoeae*

    **B.** *Chlamydia trachomatis*

    **C.** *Treponema pallidum*

    **D.** *Gardnerella vaginalis*

    **E.** *Haemophilus ducreyi*

**128.** The treatment of choice for this infection is
  **A.** doxycycline
  **B.** penicillin
  **C.** metronidazole
  **D.** trimethoprin-sulfamethoxazole
  **E.** gentamicin

**129.** Treatment for Reiter's syndrome with its triad of urethritis, conjunctivitis, and arthritis could include all of the following **EXCEPT**
  **A.** systemic steroids
  **B.** nonsteroidal anti-inflammatory drugs
  **C.** analgesics
  **D.** cytotoxic drugs
  **E.** antibiotics

**Questions 130–133:**
Match the symptoms or treatment with the disease.

  **A.** Reiter's syndrome
  **B.** gonoccocal arthritis
  **C.** both of the above

**130.** Characterized by the presence of conjunctivitis

**131.** Characterized by the presence of balanitis

**132.** More likely to affect the upper extremities

**133.** Responds to penicillin

**134.** Which of the following is the most frequently reported AIDS-defining illness?
  **A.** Invasive cervical carcinoma
  **B.** *Pneumocystis carinii* pneumonia
  **C.** HIV wasting syndrome
  **D.** Candida infections
  **E.** Kaposi's sarcoma

**Questions 135 and 136:**
Match the following.

    **A.** encouraging use of clean needles among intravenous drug users
    **B.** stressing condom usage and safer sexual practices

**135.** Choose the control method that would be most appropriate to control the AIDS epidemic in New York

**136.** Choose the control method that is most appropriate to control the AIDS epidemic in Southeast Asia.

**137.** Of the following, which is the most rapidly *increasing* cause of years of potential life lost?
    **A.** Unintentional injuries
    **B.** HIV or AIDS
    **C.** Prematurity
    **D.** Cancer
    **E.** Congenital anomalies

**138.** All of the following are part of the new Center for Disease Control and Prevention 1993 AIDS Surveillance **EXCEPT**
    **A.** invasive cervical carcinoma
    **B.** CD4-positive T-lymphocyte percentage of total lymphocytes <14
    **C.** a second episode of vaginal yeast infection
    **D.** pulmonary tuberculosis
    **E.** CD4-positive T-lymphocyte count of $<200/mm^3$

**139.** HIV infection has been most clearly *associated* with each of the following neoplastic conditions **EXCEPT**
    **A.** Kaposi's sarcoma
    **B.** non-Hodgkin's lymphoma
    **C.** squamous cell carcinoma of the anus
    **D.** invasive cervical carcinoma
    **E.** endometrial carcinoma

**140.** In 1993 the number of cases of AIDS attributed to heterosexual transmission to an uninfected partner was highest in which of the following groups?
   **A.** Intravenous drug users
   **B.** Transfusion recipients
   **C.** Persons with hemophilia
   **D.** Bisexual men
   **E.** Rape victims

**141.** The following symptoms are common in *Salmonella typhi* infection **EXCEPT**
   **A.** fever
   **B.** chill
   **C.** malaise
   **D.** diarrhea
   **E.** vomiting

**142.** Effective treatment of *Salmonella typhi* includes the following **EXCEPT**
   **A.** chloramphenicol
   **B.** trimethoprim–sulfamethoxazole (Septra)
   **C.** ampicillin
   **D.** ketoconazole
   **E.** ciprofloxacin

**143.** The following are true concerning *Vibrio cholerae* **EXCEPT**
   **A.** protein endotoxin
   **B.** water is its primary vehicle of infection
   **C.** bloody diarrhea
   **D.** noninvasive
   **E.** rehydration is crucial

**144.** The following are *bacterial* causes of gastrointestinal infection **EXCEPT**
   **A.** salmonella
   **B.** shigella
   **C.** *Yersinia entercolitica*
   **D.** *Giardia lamblia*
   **E.** *Vibrio cholerae*

**145.** Which of the following is **NOT** true concerning *Legionella*?
A. Transmitted by water droplets, especially from water coolers
B. Drug of choice is erythromycin
C. Transmissible from person to person
D. Older persons at greater risk
E. Patients who smoke or have chronic pulmonary disease are more susceptible

**146.** Which of the following is **NOT** true concerning *Giardia lamblia*?
A. Humans are the main reservoirs
B. Day care centers are commonly affected
C. Transmitted by fecal-oral route
D. Amphotericin is the drug of choice
E. Chlorination does not kill the cysts

**147.** Which of the following is true about staphylococcal food poisoning?
A. Toxin is heat-labile
B. Onset is gradual
C. Staphylococci are usually found in high concentrations in contaminated food
D. Foods rich in protein and handled often are primarily affected (custards, cream fillings, and sliced meats)
E. Recovery is slow—greater than 12 to 24 hours

**148.** Which is **NOT** true of salmonella food poisoning?
A. Incubation is usually 72 to 96 hours
B. Diarrhea is usually present
C. Primary source is raw meat, meat products, dairy products, and eggs
D. Poultry is affected more commonly than beef
E. *Salmonella* is a gram-negative bacillus

**149.** The following drugs are effective against *Salmonella typhi* **EXCEPT**
A. chloramphenicol
B. ampicillin
C. trimethaprim-sulfamethoxazole
D. erythromycin
E. ceftriaxone

**150.** Which of the following is **NOT** a potential cause of *Clostridium perfringens* food poisoning?
  **A.** Cooking meat in large quantities
  **B.** Prolonged storage at room temperature
  **C.** Rapid cooling of food
  **D.** Inadequate reheating of food
  **E.** Contamination of meat by flies and dust

**151.** Which of the following is true concerning botulism?
  **A.** *Clostridium botulinum* is a gram-positive, aerobic bacillus
  **B.** Symptoms are caused by a preformed toxin
  **C.** The toxin is heat-stable
  **D.** Most outbreaks are due to commercial canning
  **E.** Disease frequently occurs with wounds contaminated with *Clostridium botulinum*

**152.** Which of the following is **NOT** true concerning food poisoning from *Vibrio parahaemolyticus*?
  **A.** It is the leading cause of food poisoning in Japan
  **B.** Primary source is crustaceans from warm coastal waters
  **C.** Incubation time is about 2 to 4 hours
  **D.** It causes salmonellosis-like symptoms
  **E.** The number of cases of *V. parahaemolyticus* infection increases during the summer months

**153.** All of the following are associated with seafood poisoning **EXCEPT**
  **A.** *Vibrio parahaemolyticus*
  **B.** ciguatera
  **C.** red tide
  **D.** *Proteus morganii*
  **E.** *Yersinia enterocolitica*

**154.** Appropriate treatment of *Shigella* infections include the following **EXCEPT**
  **A.** trimethoprim-sulfamethoxazole
  **B.** ampicillin
  **C.** norfloxacin
  **D.** anti-diarrheal agents
  **E.** ciprofloxacin

**155.** The usual order of incidence (highest to lowest) of nosocomial infections in US hospitals is

    **A.** lower respiratory tract, urinary tract, surgical wound, bloodstream

    **B.** urinary tract, lower respiratory tract, surgical wound, bloodstream

    **C.** lower respiratory tract, urinary tract, bloodstream, surgical wound

    **D.** urinary tract, surgical wound, lower respiratory tract, bloodstream

    **E.** bloodstream, surgical wound, urinary tract, lower respiratory tract

**Questions 156–158:**
Choose the **BEST** answer for each.

    **A.** *Legionella pneumophila*
    **B.** *Streptococcus pneumoniae*
    **C.** *Candida*
    **D.** enterococci
    **E.** *Klebsiella pneumoniae*

**156.** One of the top three nosocomial bloodstream pathogens

**157.** Causes sporadic and occasionally epidemic lower respiratory tract infections in certain hospitals

**158.** An important nonbacterial cause of bloodstream infections in patients on chemotherapy

**Questions 159 and 160:**
Choose the **BEST** answer for each.

    **A.** *Haemophilus influenzae*
    **B.** hepatitis A virus
    **C.** cytomegalovirus
    **D.** *Shigella*
    **E.** scabies

**159.** A symptomatic infection that frequently affects children, day-care staff, and close family members, especially siblings.

**160.** Infection is inapparent in children attending day-care facilities but is likely to be significant in their adult contacts.

**161.** Regarding epidemic typhus, all of the following are true **EXCEPT**
   **A.** it is present in remote areas of Africa
   **B.** overcrowding, poverty, and infrequent bathing are contributing social factors
   **C.** fever, chills, and faint macular rash over the trunk are common
   **D.** erythromycin is usually curative and is the treatment of choice
   **E.** man is the host and long-term reservoir

**162.** Regarding scrub typhus, all of the following are true **EXCEPT**
   **A.** mostly self-limiting if untreated
   **B.** seen in hot, wet tropical climates
   **C.** life cycle involves larval mites (chiggers)
   **D.** doxycycline is particularly reliable
   **E.** first sign of disease is a vesicle followed by an eschar in 90% of patients

**163.** Rickettsial infections are associated with all of the following **EXCEPT**
   **A.** obligate intracellular parasite
   **B.** severe headaches, fever, myalgia, and rash
   **C.** trench fever and Brill-Zinsser disease
   **D.** transmission to humans primarily by direct salivary inoculation through biting
   **E.** various ticks included among vectors and major hosts

**164.** Which of the following is most closely associated with Q fever?
   **A.** Maculopapular rash
   **B.** Limited to the Western Hemisphere
   **C.** Insecticide spraying of cattle, sheep, and goats possible effective control
   **D.** Formaldehyde vaccine commercially available
   **E.** Person-to-person transmission common

**Questions 165–167:**
Match the following.

  A. human body louse
  B. no rash
  C. Western Hemisphere

**165.** Q fever

**166.** Trench fever

**167.** Rocky Mountain spotted fever

**168.** Select the best answer regarding human plague.
  A. Penicillin is effective and is the treatment of choice
  B. Fever, chills, and lymph node pain occur within 7 days
  C. Diagnosis is best made with serologic tests
  D. Mode of transmission is fecal-oral
  E. The classic clinical form of the disease is meningial

**169.** The infected female *Anopheles* mosquito inoculates malarial sporozoites into a human while feeding. Within 30 minutes, these sporozoites
  A. enter RBCs
  B. enter hepatocytes
  C. become schizonts
  D. release merozoites
  E. release gametes

**170.** Ideally, the diagnosis of malaria in a febrile patient is confirmed by
  A. serologic testing
  B. liver biopsy
  C. identification of malaria parasites on a blood smear (Giemsa stain)
  D. fever, chills, and sweats in a person with no prior exposure to the parasite
  E. monitoring fever pattern

**171.** Which of the following species of *Plasmodium* causes the most deaths?

    **A.** *P. falciparum*
    **B.** *P. vivax*
    **C.** *P. malariae*
    **D.** *P. ovale*
    **E.** *P. quintana*

**172.** Placental malaria infection is commonly associated with each of the following **EXCEPT**

    **A.** severe anemia
    **B.** low birth weight
    **C.** premature birth
    **D.** toxemia
    **E.** acute pulmonary edema

**173.** The most drug-resistant malarial parasites in the world are currently found in

    **A.** sub-Sahara Africa
    **B.** regions of Thailand and Burma
    **C.** Amazon region of Brazil
    **D.** the Middle East
    **E.** Panama Canal Zone

**Questions 174–177:**
Match the following organisms and diseases.

    **A.** Q fever
    **B.** plague
    **C.** Rocky Mountain spotted fever
    **D.** epidemic typus

**174.** *Yersinia pestis*

**175.** *Coxiella burnetii*

**176.** *Rickettsia prowazekii*

**177.** *Rickettsia rickettsii*

**178.** All of the following diseases are transmitted by ticks **EXCEPT**
A. epidemic typhus
B. Rocky Mountain spotted fever
C. Relapsing fever
D. Lyme disease
E. Mediterranean spotted fever

**179.** A 21-year-old man comes to your office with painful, tender, enlarged, draining left inguinal nodes of 2 days' duration. He also complains of chills, fever, malaise, nausea, and pains in the limbs and back. He has just returned from a trip to Vietnam. The most likely diagnosis is
A. lymphadenopathy of cat-scratch fever
B. bubonic plague
C. tularemia
D. lymphogranuloma venereum
E. suppurative gonorrhea

**180.** Which is **NOT** an appropriate antibiotic for the treatment of *Yersinia pestis*?
A. Streptomycin
B. Chloramphenicol
C. Tetracycline
D. Penicillin
E. Sulfadiazine

**181.** Which of the following is **NOT** a mosquito-borne viral infection?
A. Eastern equine encephalitis
B. Yellow fever
C. St. Louis encephalitis
D. Malaria
E. Western equine encephalitis

**182.** Which of the following organisms has **NOT** developed significant antibiotic resistance in recent years?
A. *Mycobacterium tuberculosis*
B. *Treponema pallidum*
C. *Staphylococcus aureus*
D. *Enterococcus faecium* (enterococcus)
E. *Streptococcus pneumoniae* (pneumococcus)

**183.** A 20% increase in reported cases of tuberculosis in the United States since the early 1980s has been attributed to all of the following factors **EXCEPT**
   **A.** the HIV epidemic
   **B.** immigration from countries whose tuberculosis incidence rates are 10 to 30 times higher than in the United States
   **C.** more highly infectious strains of drug-resistant tuberculosis circulating in the United States during these years
   **D.** declines in resources for tuberculosis control
   **E.** continued overcrowding in nursing homes, correctional institutions, and homeless shelters

**184.** Ebola virus infection identified in outbreaks of viral hemorrhagic fever in Zaire and Sudan in 1976 and in Zaire in 1995 has been characterized by which of the following?
   **A.** Predominance of airborne transmission by coughing individuals
   **B.** Generalized persistent lymphadenopathy
   **C.** Severe polyarthritis
   **D.** Mortality rates of at least 50%
   **E.** At least 80% preventability by EVV (Ebola virus vaccine)

**185.** Under the expanded adult and adolescent AIDS case definition for surveillance purposes that has been used by the Centers for Disease Control and Prevention since 1993, which one of the following findings in an HIV-infected individual is sufficient to define the case as acquired immunodeficiency syndrome?
   **A.** Persistent generalized lymphadenopathy
   **B.** CD4 lymphocyte count of under 200 per $mm^3$
   **C.** Recurrent bronchitis in a 12-month period
   **D.** Cervical dysplasia
   **E.** Oral candidiasis

**186.** Which of the following is true regarding chlamydial infection in the United States?
   **A.** Chlamydia is currently believed to have an incidence second only to gonorrhea as a sexually transmitted disease in the United States
   **B.** Chlamydial infection is usually clinically distinguishable from gonorrheal infection
   **C.** Treatment for gonorrheal infection should always be accompanied by presumptive treatment for chlamydial infection

**D.** Only symptomatic cases of chlamydial infection are associated with subsequent risk of infertility and ectopic pregnancy

**E.** Teenagers in rural areas are the highest risk group

**187.** All of the following have been associated with chlamydial infections, **EXCEPT**
**A.** bartholinitis
**B.** perihepatitis
**C.** conjunctival and pneumonic infection of the newborn
**D.** mucopurulent cervicitis
**E.** hepatitis

**188.** Which of the following is true regarding cryptococcosis?
**A.** Usually presents as a subacute or chronic meningitis
**B.** Untreated cryptococcal meningitis usually terminates fatally within a few days
**C.** Approximately 35% of AIDS patients in the United States and Africa have developed cryptococcosis
**D.** Responds to intravenous antibiotics
**E.** Sputum cultures are positive in 60% of cases

**189.** Which of the following is true regarding dengue fever?
**A.** The infectious agent involved in dengue fever belongs in the category of rickettsiae
**B.** Fatalities are common with this disease, even in the absence of dengue hemorrhagic fever
**C.** The mode of transmission is by the bite of infected mosquitoes
**D.** Prevention depends on the use of vaccine and postexposure immune globulin
**E.** Onset is slow and insidious

**190.** The Epstein-Barr virus has been associated with all of the following conditions **EXCEPT**
**A.** infectious mononucleosis
**B.** African Burkitt's lymphoma
**C.** nasopharyngeal cancer
**D.** primary hepatic carcinoma
**E.** acute fatal immunoblastic sarcoma in AIDS patients

**191.** Regarding the diagnosis of Epstein-Barr virus (EBV) infection, all of the following are true **EXCEPT**
  **A.** a laboratory diagnosis of EBV infection may be made after the finding of a lymphocytosis exceeding 50% (including 10% abnormal forms) and a positive heterophile antibody test
  **B.** this virus has been conclusively proven to be the cause of chronic fatigue syndrome
  **C.** among young adults with acute EBV infection, 95% will have abnormal liver function tests
  **D.** although several organisms, including cytomegalovirus and toxoplasma, may produce clinical and hematologic findings resembling EBV infection, only EBV elicits the heterophile antibody
  **E.** an infrequent complication is autoimmune hemolytic anemia

**192.** Regarding echinococcosis, which of the following is **CORRECT?**
  **A.** The etiologic agent is a tapeworm
  **B.** There are four different clinical manifestations, caused by four closely related species
  **C.** The lesions can be defined by CT scanning and sonography, but not by roentgenography
  **D.** The dog, wolf, dingo, and other Canidae are the usual intermediate hosts
  **E.** The primary susceptible group is dry land grain farmers

**193.** The World Health Assembly has adopted a resolution to eliminate dracunculiasis (guinea worm infection) from the world in the 1990s. All of the following are correct regarding dracunculiasis **EXCEPT**
  **A.** the infection is caused by a large tapeworm
  **B.** the female organism, after mating, migrates to the subcutaneous tissues (most frequently of the legs)
  **C.** eosinophilia in an afflicted person may appear around the time of vesicle formation
  **D.** the incubation period is usually about 12 months
  **E.** all of the above

**194.** All of the following are true regarding hookworm disease **EXCEPT**
  **A.** iron-deficiency anemia is the major cause of disability from the disease
  **B.** it can be associated with retarded mental and physical development in children

C. light hookworm infections generally produce clinical effects
D. hookworm is primarily a problem of developing countries
E. poor sanitation is the major contributing cause of the disease

**195.** All of the following are true regarding clonorchiasis **EXCEPT**
    **A.** a chronic disease, sometimes of 30 years or longer duration, often completely asymptomatic
    **B.** a significant risk factor for development of cholangiocarcinoma
    **C.** infection caused by eating raw or undercooked freshwater fish or crayfish
    **D.** man is the only known reservoir of the disease
    **E.** the treatment of choice is praziquantel

**196.** All of the following are true with regard to hepatitis C infection **EXCEPT**
    **A.** it progresses to jaundice less frequently than hepatitis B infection
    **B.** chronic infection may progress to cirrhosis
    **C.** diagnostic serologic test is designed to detect surface antigen of the virus
    **D.** it is the most common post-transfusion hepatitis in the United States
    **E.** it is believed to have been the leading cause of transfusion-associated hepatitis in the 1970s and 1980s

**197.** All of the following are true regarding human papillomavirus (HPV) infection **EXCEPT**
    **A.** HPV types 16 and 18 have been associated with cervical neoplasia
    **B.** HPV types 6 and 11 have been associated with genital warts and laryngeal papillomata
    **C.** Condyloma acuminatum is usually sexually transmitted
    **D.** the cause of laryngeal papillomata is probably transmitted during passage of the infant through the birth canal
    **E.** HPV is an RNA virus, closely related to the hepatitis A virus

**198.** Regarding leprosy, which of the following is true?

  **A.** A more socially acceptable name for leprosy is Harris' disease

  **B.** The two classically described clinical manifestations of the disease are lepromatous and granulomatous or tuberculoid leprosy

  **C.** The diagnosis of lepromatous leprosy is strongly supported by demonstrating acid-fast bacilli in skin smears

  **D.** The etiologic organism is *Leprobacterium leprae*

  **E.** All of the different treatment regimens recommended by the World Health Organization call for prolonged treatment with a single drug

**199.** Which of the following is true regarding Lyme disease?

  **A.** The usual first clinical manifestation is a distinctive skin rash

  **B.** Serologic tests for the etiologic agent are usually very sensitive during the first several weeks of the infection

  **C.** For adults, the current first-line treatment recommendation is to use high-dose erythromycin for 2 to 5 days

  **D.** The causative organism is an arbovirus

  **E.** Antibiotic treatment in the early stages of the illness does not prevent chronic illness

**200.** All of the following are true regarding erythema infectiosum (fifth disease) **EXCEPT**

  **A.** the etiologic agent is echovirus B19

  **B.** the etiologic agent is parvovirus B19

  **C.** the etiologic agent responsible for erythema infectiosum has also been associated with transient aplastic crises in patients with chronic hemolytic diseases

  **D.** characteristic of this disease is a slapped-cheek appearance followed by a lace-like rash on the trunk and extremities

  **E.** epidemics involving school-age children often occur

**201.** Regarding gonorrhea, all of the following are true **EXCEPT**

  **A.** the Centers for Disease Control (CDC) recommends that all gonorrhea cases should be diagnosed or confirmed by culture

  **B.** the CDC's recommendation for first-line therapy of uncomplicated urethral, endocervical, or rectal gonorrhea includes ceftriaxone as well as doxycycline for possible concurrent chlamydial infection

    **C.** CDC recommends that all patents with gonorrhea should have a serologic test for syphilis and should be offered confidential counseling and testing for HIV infection

    **D.** CDC recommends that pregnant women should be cultured for *Neisseria gonorrhoeae* (and tested for *Chlamydia trachomatis* and syphilis) at the first prenatal-care visit

    **E.** CDC does not recommend the use of ceftriaxone to treat gonococcal infections in pregnancy because of its possible effects on the fetus

**202.** All of the following statements about *Haemophilus influenzae* type B (Hib) vaccines are correct **EXCEPT**

    **A.** the Advisory Committee on Immunization Practices recommends that all children receive a series of vaccinations with one of the conjugate vaccines licensed for infant use, beginning routinely at 2 months of age

    **B.** unvaccinated children 15 to 59 months of age may be given a single dose of any of the conjugate vaccines

    **C.** the currently licensed vaccines do not all follow the same age schedules for the immunization series

    **D.** it is recommended that the same conjugate vaccine should be used throughout the vaccination series

    **E.** Hib conjugate vaccines should not be given simultaneously with live virus vaccines such as measles-mumps-rubella (MMR) or oral polio vaccine (OPV)

**203.** Regarding hepatitis B infection, all of the following are true **EXCEPT**

    **A.** it is caused by an RNA virus

    **B.** hepatitis B surface antibody (anti-HBs) develops after a resolved infection and is believed to be responsible for long-term immunity

    **C.** antibody to core antigen (anti-HBc) develops in all HBV infections and persists indefinitely, regardless of recovery or immunity

    **D.** IgM anti-HBc appears early in infection and persists for up to approximately 6 months

    **E.** infants infected with HBV at birth have a 90% chance of becoming chronic carriers

**204.** Worldwide, hepatitis B infection is associated with all of the following **EXCEPT**
  **A.** acute hepatitis
  **B.** chronic hepatitis
  **C.** cirrhosis
  **D.** primary hepatocellular carcinoma
  **E.** cancer of the gallbladder

**205.** A patient is found to be positive for hepatitis B core antibody (anti-HBc) but negative for hepatitis B surface antibody (anti-HBs). All of the following responses are true **EXCEPT**
  **A.** the patient could be a carrier of hepatitis B
  **B.** the patient's status could be clarified by testing for hepatitis B surface antigen (HBsAg) and IgM hepatitis B core antibody
  **C.** the patient has been exposed to hepatitis B in the past but has recovered and is now immune
  **D.** the patient could be in the "core window" of the recovery phase of an acute hepatitis B infection
  **E.** the patient's anti-HBc could *not* have been caused by hepatitis B immunization

**206.** Concerning the epidemiology of acquired immunodeficiency syndrome (AIDS) and human immunodeficiency virus (HIV) infection in the United States, all of the following are true **EXCEPT**
  **A.** AIDS is now among the leading causes of death among men 25 to 44 years of age in the United States
  **B.** AIDS is now one of the ten leading causes of death among women 15 to 44 years of age in the United States
  **C.** the World Health Organization estimated in 1991 that 8 to 10 million adults and 1 million children worldwide were infected with the HIV
  **D.** the World Health Organization estimated in 1991 that by the year 2000, 40 million persons may be infected with HIV
  **E.** worldwide, most persons with HIV infection reside in developed countries with high rates of intravenous drug abuse and homosexual activity

**207.** Concerning the epidemiology of AIDS in the United States, all of the following are true **EXCEPT**
   **A.** AIDS cases in homosexual and bisexual men and intravenous drug users have accounted for the largest number of cases throughout the epidemic but are now decreasing
   **B.** AIDS cases associated with heterosexual transmission of HIV have been increasing steadily
   **C.** AIDS cases associated with heterosexual transmission of HIV are occurring more frequently among women than men
   **D.** AIDS cases in children associated with perinatal (mother-to-infant) HIV transmission have continued to increase
   **E.** the number of new AIDS cases associated with blood or blood product transfusions continues to rise annually

**208.** Which of these is the most common opportunistic infection associated with AIDS?
   **A.** Kaposi's sarcoma
   **B.** HIV encephalopathy
   **C.** Esophageal candidiasis
   **D.** *Pneumocystis carinii* pneumonia
   **E.** Cytomegalovirus retinitis

**209.** In areas where travelers will be at risk of acquiring chloroquine-resistant *Plasmodium falciparum* malaria, which of the following is the drug of choice for prophylaxis?
   **A.** Primaquine
   **B.** Sulfadoxine-pyrimethamine (Fansidar)
   **C.** Quinine
   **D.** Quinidine
   **E.** Mefloquine

**210.** For malaria cases involving grave infection, the therapy of choice is immediate treatment with which of the following?
   **A.** Chloroquine
   **B.** Primaquine
   **C.** Sulfadoxine-pyrimethamine (Fansidar)
   **D.** Quinine or quinidine
   **E.** Mefloquine

**211.** Which of the following is the drug of choice for treating methicillin-resistant *Staphylococcus aureus* (MRSA) infections?
**A.** Erythromycin
**B.** Vancomycin
**C.** Tetracycline
**D.** Aminoglycosides
**E.** Trimethoprim-sulfamethosoxazole

**212.** Concerning infection with *Mycobacterium tuberculosis,* which of the following is true?
**A.** In 40% of patients, initial infection may progress directly to pulmonary tuberculosis
**B.** BCG vaccination should be considered for use in all HIV-infected patients because of their high risk of TB
**C.** In persons with HIV infection, a PPD test with as little as 5 mm of induration should be considered indicative of tuberculous infection
**D.** Extrapulmonary tuberculosis is now nearly as common as pulmonary in the United States
**E.** The incidence of drug-resistant TB has been decreasing in the United States over the past 5 to 10 years

**213.** Which of the following is the **INCORRECT** statement concerning mycobacterial infection in persons with HIV infection?
**A.** The most common mycobacterial species isolated from patients with diagnosed AIDS are *Mycobacterium avium intracellulare* and *M. kansasii*
**B.** Clinicians should consider the diagnosis of tuberculosis in patients with (or at risk of) HIV infection even if the clinical presentation is unusual
**C.** Pulmonary tuberculosis in patients with HIV infection is easily distinguished from other pulmonary infections such as *Pneumocystis carinii* pneumonia
**D.** Chemotherapy should be started whenever acid-fast bacilli are found in a specimen from a patient with HIV infection and there is clinical evidence of mycobacterial disease
**E.** Individuals who are known to be HIV-positive should be given a Mantoux skin test with five tuberculin units of PPD as part of their clinical evaluation

**214.** Cases of botulism in humans in the United States are classified into four categories. Which of the following is the **INCORRECT** category?

A. Pulmonary botulism
B. Food-borne botulism
C. Infant botulism
D. Wound botulism
E. Undetermined classification

**215.** Foods implicated in outbreaks of botulism have included all of the following **EXCEPT**

A. vegetables (such as chili peppers)
B. fruits (such as low-acid tomatoes)
C. meats
D. honey
E. avocados

**216.** Which of the following is **INCORRECT** concerning infant botulism?

A. In the typical case, the child is about 3 months old
B. The first symptom is usually constipation
C. The infant typically appears "floppy"
D. The fatality rate for cases requiring hospitalization in the United States is over 20%
E. Some cases of sudden infant death syndrome might be attributable to infant botulism

**217.** Which is **INCORRECT** concerning subacute sclerosing panencephalitis (SSPE)?

A. Is a rare complication of measles which may result in permanent sequelae
B. Mean incubation period is 7 years from measles illness
C. Measles vaccine, by protecting against measles, significantly reduces the possibility of developing SSPE
D. SSPE in children with no history of natural measles but a history of receiving measles vaccine has been reported
E. Rubella virus has been implicated as a triggering factor

**218.** All of the following are true concerning poliovirus **EXCEPT**
  **A.** oral polio virus vaccine (OPV) is a live-virus vaccine
  **B.** parenterally administered polio virus vaccine (IPV) is a killed-virus vaccine
  **C.** measles-mumps-rubella (MMR) vaccine and OPV should not be given simultaneously
  **D.** adults who have not been adequately immunized against poliomyelitis with OPV or IPV are at a minimal risk of developing OPV-associated paralytic poliomyelitis when children in the household or day care facility in which they work are given OPV
  **E.** a minimum interval of 6 weeks between OPV doses, usually 2 months, is recommended

**219.** All of the following are true concerning oral poliomyelitis vaccine **EXCEPT**
  **A.** the vaccine offers 95% 100% protection against poliovirus
  **B.** as a result of this vaccine, disease caused by wild poliovirus has been virtually eliminated in the United States
  **C.** one out of every 2.6 million vaccine doses results in paralytic poliomyelitis
  **D.** most cases of endemic poliomyelitis in the United States since 1981 (about eight cases per year) have been associated with the vaccine
  **E.** the World Health Organization has plans to eradicate polio worldwide by the year 2025

**220.** All of the following concerning pneumococcal pneumonia are true **EXCEPT**
  **A.** accounts for over half of all pneumonias
  **B.** associated with high rates of bacteremia in the very young and very old
  **C.** current case fatality rate is only half of rate prior to effective antimicrobial therapy
  **D.** multivalent pneumococcal vaccine is highly protective
  **E.** most cases are community-acquired

**221.** Which of the following is **INCORRECT** concerning pneumococcal vaccine?
   **A.** Composed of purified polysaccharide capsular antigens
   **B.** Not recommended for use in patients with HIV infection
   **C.** Not recommended for use in children under 2 years of age
   **D.** Recommended for patients with nephrotic syndrome
   **E.** Recommended for healthy older adults, together with influenza vaccine

**222.** Concerning Legionnaire's disease and the organism *Legionella pneumophila*, what is the **INCORRECT** statement?
   **A.** Occurs in both epidemic and sporadic form
   **B.** Has an estimated incidence of 25,000 to 50,000 cases yearly in the United States
   **C.** Is rarely isolated from water sources unrelated to outbreaks of human disease
   **D.** Is not identified by routine testing of potable water systems or cooling towers for the causative agent, *L. pneumophila*
   **E.** In epidemic form, usually results from exposure of susceptible individuals to an aerosol generated by an environmental source of water contaminated with *Legionella*

**223.** Identify the **INCORRECT** statement concerning health information for international travel.
   **A.** Some countries require an international certificate of vaccination against yellow fever as a condition for entry
   **B.** Most US international travelers do not need additional immunizations, provided their routine immunization status is up to date
   **C.** Data on the occurrence of many communicable diseases, as published by the World Health Organization (WHO), are considered nearly complete and correct
   **D.** Travelers visiting tourist areas on itineraries that do not include visits to rural areas have minimal risk of exposure to food or water of questionable quality
   **E.** Depending on the areas being visited, additional recommended vaccines may include polio, meningitis, or typhoid

**224.** Identify the **INCORRECT** statement concerning the use of different vaccines.
   **A.** Inactivated vaccines should *not* be administered simultaneously
   **B.** Most live-virus vaccines may be administered on the same day without impairing antibody response
   **C.** Live-virus vaccines that are not administered on the same day should be given at least 1 month apart
   **D.** An inactivated vaccine and a live-attenuated-virus vaccine may be administered simultaneously at different sites
   **E.** None of the above

**225.** Sometimes it is necessary to protect a patient with immune globulin (Ig). Which of the statements below concerning immune globulin is **INCORRECT**?
   **A.** Inactivated products can be given any time after Ig use
   **B.** With live attenuated vaccines, immune globulin may interfere with production of vaccine antibodies
   **C.** Live vaccines (eg, MMR) should *not* be given for at least 2 weeks before Ig and for at least 6 weeks after the administration of Ig
   **D.** If the interval between vaccine and Ig is less than 14 days, the vaccine should be repeated
   **E.** It is never safe to administer Ig and live-virus vaccine simultaneously

**226.** Advice for travelers to malaria endemic areas could include each of the following **EXCEPT**
   **A.** all travelers to malarious areas of the world are advised to take an appropriate drug regimen to prevent malaria
   **B.** travelers can be advised that if an appropriate drug regimen is taken, they are safe from the likelihood of contracting malaria
   **C.** persons who develop symptoms of malaria should seek prompt medical evaluation, including thick and thin malaria smears, as soon as possible
   **D.** malaria symptoms can develop as early as 8 days after initial exposure
   **E.** malaria symptoms can appear months after departure from a malarious area, after chemoprophylaxis is discontinued

**227.** Influenza is one of the greatest pandemic diseases because of
    **A.** mutation of the virus
    **B.** spread by water
    **C.** long incubation period
    **D.** high fatality rate
    **E.** lack of specific vaccines

**228.** Schistosomiasis, or bilharziasis, is a helminthic infection of the mesenteric, portal, and pelvic venous systems. At least 150 million people are currently infected. Effective control has been rare. The vector involved is
    **A.** man
    **B.** fish
    **C.** snails
    **D.** mosquitoes
    **E.** cercariae

**229.** Control measures for schistosomiasis include
    **A.** reduction of snail population
    **B.** raising and lowering water levels
    **C.** DDT for mosquitoes
    **D.** spraying of sodium pentachlorophenate to kill infected fish
    **E.** treatment of known cases

**230.** The primary mode of transmission of tuberculosis is
    **A.** airborne
    **B.** fomites
    **C.** arthropods
    **D.** flies
    **E.** direct invasion through breaks in the skin

**231.** In a patient found to have bubonic plague
    **A.** the definitive diagnosis would have been made on the basis of blood culture
    **B.** he should receive the vaccine at once
    **C.** the most effective antibiotic is erythromycin
    **D.** the period of incubation is 2 to 7 days
    **E.** quarantine of the patient is not advisable

**232.** *Vibrio cholerae* proliferates within the lumen of the intestine and
   A. invades the bloodstream
   B. invades the tissues
   C. inhibits sodium transport
   D. produces little effect on electrolytes
   E. allows resorption of isotonic fluids

**233.** The virus most often associated with colds in adults is
   A. rhinovirus
   B. coxsackievirus
   C. echovirus
   D. respiratory syncytial virus (RSV)
   E. parainfluenza virus

**234.** All of the following are true of fungi **EXCEPT**
   A. only the dermatophytes and *Candida* are commonly transmitted from one human to another
   B. pathogenic fungi generally produce no toxins
   C. in systemic mycoses, the typical tissue reaction is a chronic granuloma
   D. the organisms responsible for tinea pedis (athlete's foot) belong to the *Microsporum* genus
   E. *Trichophyton corporis* usually affects the areas of nonhairy, smooth skin

**235.** All of the following diseases are transmitted by contact (direct, indirect, or droplets) **EXCEPT**
   A. anthrax
   B. ascariasis
   C. chickenpox
   D. gonorrhea
   E. smallpox

**236.** All of the following are characteristics of staphylococcal food poisoning **EXCEPT**
   A. symptoms usually begin 2 to 4 hours after ingestion
   B. the onset of symptoms is abrupt
   C. patient's temperature is usually 101° to 102°F
   D. fatalities in normal individuals are rare
   E. diarrhea, if present, may be severe

**237.** Influenza is characterized epidemiologically by all of the following **EXCEPT**
  A. epidemic-pandemic potentiality
  B. excess mortality among predictable high-risk groups
  C. high morbidity and low mortality
  D. periodic-cyclic recurrences
  E. in the temperate zones, epidemics tend to occur in the late summer

**238.** Which of the following does **NOT** require complete or modified quarantine for specific protection?
  A. Diphtheria
  B. Hepatitis A
  C. Typhoid fever
  D. Pemphigus neonatorum
  E. Malaria

**239.** Which type of malaria is characterized by a 48-hour developmental cycle, cerebral symptoms, biliary remittent fever, shock, hemoglobinuria?
  A. *Plasmodium falciparum*
  B. *P. vivax*
  C. *P. malariae*
  D. *P. ovale*
  E. A rare combination of *P. vivax* and *P. ovale*

**240.** All of the following are true concerning meningococcal meningitis **EXCEPT**
  A. there are no limits in geographic distribution
  B. it occurs in men more than women
  C. it occurs more commonly in adults under crowded living conditions, such as in barracks and institutions
  D. the greatest prevalence is during winter and spring
  E. the reservoir is equestrian

**241.** Which of the following is **INCORRECT** concerning leptospirosis?
  **A.** Leptospirosis is a zoonotic disease caused by any of a large number of spirochetes
  **B.** A common clinical feature is severe myalgia, especially of the calves and thighs
  **C.** Cases are often misdiagnosed as meningitis or encephalitis
  **D.** The case fatality rate is generally high
  **E.** Diagnosis is confirmed by rising titers in serologic tests

**242.** Which of the following is **INCORRECT** concerning mechanisms for transmission of leptospirosis?
  **A.** Contact of the skin with water contaminated with the urine of infected animals can transmit the disease
  **B.** Direct contact with urine or tissues of infected animals can transmit the disease
  **C.** Ingestion of food contaminated with urine of infected rats can transmit the disease
  **D.** Inhalation of droplet aerosols of contaminated fluids can occasionally transmit the disease
  **E.** Direct person-to-person transmission is quite common

**243.** Concerning yellow fever and its vaccine, which is **INCORRECT**?
  **A.** Active immunization is appropriate for all persons over 9 months of age who are necessarily exposed to infection because of residence, occupation, or travel
  **B.** A single, subcutaneous injection of a vaccine containing live attenuated virus is effective in almost 99% of recipients
  **C.** Revaccination every 10 years is required by the International Health Regulations for travel from endemic areas
  **D.** Pronounced leukocytosis occurs early in the disease, particularly in the first week
  **E.** Jaundice is moderate early in the disease and is intensified later

**Questions 244–246:**
Three members of a family of eight are admitted to the hospital with similar findings: nausea, vomiting, abdominal cramps, sudden edema of the eyelids, subconjunctival hemorrhages, and photophobia. Each complains of muscle soreness and pain with chills and fever. Two have transient neurologic signs and one develops myocarditis. The family lives on

the outskirts of town on a farm. They grow and home-can most of their fruits and vegetables. Their meat supply is obtained from farm hogs, chickens, and hunted wildlife.

**244.** The most likely diagnosis is
 **A.** dermatomyositis
 **B.** ascaris infestation
 **C.** trichinosis
 **D.** schistosomiasis
 **E.** salmonellosis

**245.** Which of the following would be the most definitive diagnostic test for these ill patients?
 **A.** Blood cultures
 **B.** Eosinophil count
 **C.** Muscle biopsy
 **D.** Stools for ova and parasites
 **E.** Serial antibody titers

**246.** The disease could have been prevented by
 **A.** ensuring that meat and meat products are federally inspected
 **B.** rodent control
 **C.** prophylactic active immunization
 **D.** quarantining the patients
 **E.** sufficiently cooking ingested meat

**Questions 247–249:**
This disease is an acute, specific infection of the alimentary tract. The onset may be with moderate diarrhea, increasing in severity, but more frequently is with sudden violent diarrhea and vomiting. The typical finding is rice-water stools.

**247.** The most likely disease involved is
 **A.** ascariasis
 **B.** giardia
 **C.** typhus
 **D.** typhoid fever
 **E.** cholera

**248.** The usual modes of transmission include all of the following **EXCEPT**
  **A.** infected food
  **B.** infected water
  **C.** fecal-oral spread
  **D.** milk
  **E.** flies

**Questions 249 and 250:**
A man returned from a hunting trip in northern California and found a tick clinging to his scalp. He removed the tick. About 4 days later he presented with the following symptoms: headache, chills, fever, and vomiting. The site of the tick bite was ulcerated; regional lymph nodes were enlarged. No rash was noted.

**249.** The most likely diagnosis is
  **A.** Rocky Mountain spotted fever
  **B.** tularemia
  **C.** relapsing fever
  **D.** plague
  **E.** dengue fever

**250.** Vectors and mechanisms known for transmitting the disease to humans include all of the following **EXCEPT**
  **A.** ticks
  **B.** person-to-person transmission
  **C.** flies
  **D.** mosquitoes
  **E.** contact exposure to infectious animal tissue

**Questions 251–253:**
This disease is a mild eruptive fever, first distinguished by the German clinician Wagner in 1829. It was considered unimportant until the observation by Gregg of the serious effects of the disease on the fetus in utero.

**251.** The disease described is
  **A.** rubeola
  **B.** smallpox
  **C.** rubella
  **D.** chickenpox
  **E.** erythema nodosum

**252.** Infection of an expectant mother is most dangerous during
    **A.** the entire 9 months of pregnancy
    **B.** the middle trimester of pregnancy
    **C.** the month before conception
    **D.** the first 3 months of pregnancy
    **E.** the final weeks of pregnancy

**253.** Symptoms frequently include all of the following **EXCEPT**
    **A.** catarrhal symptoms
    **B.** vomiting and diarrhea
    **C.** coryza
    **D.** conjunctivitis
    **E.** arthritis

**Questions 254 and 255:**
A member of the city fire department is reported to the local health department as having typhoid fever. Within 10 days, 16 more firemen also are reported to have typhoid fever. The source is traced to an annual picnic attended by 40 firemen and held 2 weeks before discovery of the first case. The picnic menu consisted of frankfurters, hamburgers, lettuce and tomato salad, corn on the cob, olives, celery, bread, butter, coffee, milk, and ice cream. The milk was obtained fresh from a dairy farm adjacent to the picnic area and was stored in a 5-gal can. The water was obtained from a state-approved community well in a nearby village. Ten of the firemen who had consumed portions of all the foods and beverages and were unaffected had been in the military service within the past 5 years.

**254.** Which of the following is the most likely source of the outbreak?
    **A.** Water
    **B.** Milk
    **C.** Bread
    **D.** Corn
    **E.** Olives

**255.** As a public health officer, you should
  A. check stools of all members of the community in which the picnic area was located
  B. immediately condemn the water supply
  C. immediately condemn the pasteurizing plant
  D. interview all at the picnic to determine foods ingested and correlation with illness
  E. take blood specimens for culture from all persons attending the picnic

**Questions 256 and 257:**
A 5-year-old child in California was taken to the doctor complaining of fever and malaise; there was also sneezing, discharge from the nose, and cough. Three days after onset of symptoms, a rash appeared.

**256.** The most likely diagnosis is
  A. measles (rubeola)
  B. smallpox
  C. chickenpox
  D. rubella
  E. exanthem subitum

**257.** Which is correct concerning the morbidity and mortality of this disease in the United States?
  A. High morbidity, high mortality
  B. High morbidity, low mortality
  C. Low morbidity, high mortality
  D. Low morbidity, low mortality
  E. Low morbidity, no mortality

**258.** Besides *Mycobacterium tuberculosis,* causative agent(s) of human tuberculosis include
  A. *M. marinum*
  B. *M. leprae*
  C. *M. bovis*
  D. *M. kansasii*
  E. *M. pneumoniae*

**Questions 259–261:**
You are asked to examine a patient with the following symptoms: fever, chills, cough, and pleural pain. While you are taking a history, the patient tells you that he spent 2 days on a fossil hunt in the Bakersfield area of the Central Valley of California about 2 weeks before the onset of symptoms.

**259.** The most likely mode of transmission was
- **A.** infection through an open wound
- **B.** contact with another person
- **C.** inhalation of spores in dust or soil, or from dry vegetation
- **D.** contact with an animal
- **E.** insect bites

**260.** The most likely diagnosis is
- **A.** coccidioidomycosis
- **B.** influenza
- **C.** tick fever
- **D.** pneumonia
- **E.** tularemia

**261.** This disease infects all of the following **EXCEPT**
- **A.** humans
- **B.** cattle
- **C.** dogs
- **D.** swine
- **E.** biting insects

**262.** Which of the following can be detected by darkfield microscopic examination?
- **A.** *Gardnerella*
- **B.** *Trichomonas*
- **C.** Gonorrhea
- **D.** Syphilis
- **E.** *Chlamydia*

**263.** Regarding pertussis, all of the following are true **EXCEPT**
   **A.** approximately 90% of deaths from this disease are in children under 1 year of age
   **B.** in unimmunized populations, pertussis is among the most lethal diseases of infants and young children
   **C.** in the United States, it is recommended that the diphtheria-pertussis-tetanus (DPT) vaccine be given at 2, 4, 12, and 24 months, with a booster after the seventh birthday
   **D.** strikingly high total white blood cell (WBC) counts with a prominent lymphocytosis may be found as the whooping stage develops
   **E.** this disease is still a major problem in developing countries

**264.** Concerning the mode of transmission of meningococcal meningitis, which of the following is **INCORRECT?**
   **A.** Animal reservoirs include monkeys
   **B.** There is person-to-person transfer
   **C.** The organism dies quickly when exposed to sunlight
   **D.** There is an association of disease with crowded living conditions
   **E.** Vaccination plays little role in control of an outbreak

**265.** *Plasmodium falciparium* malaria resistance has led to which recommended protocol for prophylaxis in adults in the country of Thailand?
   **A.** Mefloquine 250 mg orally, once per week
   **B.** Proguanil 200 mg orally each day
   **C.** Doxycycline 100 mg orally each day
   **D.** Chloroquine 300 mg base orally, once per week
   **E.** Primaquine 15 mg base orally each day

**266.** A traveler returning from central Africa is suspected of having malaria despite taking appropriate chemosuppressive medication. Options for treatment could include all of the following **EXCEPT**
   **A.** Quinidine gluconate
   **B.** Chloroquine phosphate
   **C.** Pyrimethamine-sulfadoxine
   **D.** Proguanil
   **E.** Quinine

**267.** Syphilis, gonorrhea, chancroid, and granuloma inguinale are linked together because of similar
   **A.** tissue reactions
   **B.** causative agents
   **C.** symptoms
   **D.** mode of transmission
   **E.** antibiotic treatment

**268.** Early (primary and secondary) and tertiary syphilis are most alike in which of the following respects?
   **A.** Infectiousness
   **B.** Destructiveness
   **C.** Diagnostic tests and procedures used
   **D.** Use of penicillin as the antibiotic of choice
   **E.** Symptoms

**269.** Immunization can be active or passive. Which of the following immunobiologics is **NOT** used for passive immunization?
   **A.** Pooled human Ig
   **B.** Specific Ig preparations
   **C.** Antitoxin
   **D.** Specific killed (inactivated) viruses
   **E.** Anti snake venom

**270.** Immunobiologics contain the following constituents: suspending fluids, preservatives, and adjuvants. Which of the following is true concerning adjuvants?
   **A.** They are usually antibiotics
   **B.** They are usually mercurials
   **C.** They are added to prevent bacterial or viral growth
   **D.** They are usually aluminum compounds
   **E.** They are usually sulfur compounds

**271.** Which of the following is **INCORRECT** concerning vaccination during pregnancy?
  **A.** Pregnancy is a contraindication for the use of vaccines against rubella, measles, and mumps
  **B.** If a vaccine must be given during pregnancy, it is wise to wait until the second or third trimester whenever possible
  **C.** Vaccinating pregnant women with killed (inactivated) vaccine is contraindicated because of risk to the fetus
  **D.** Tetanus and diphtheria toxoid should be given to inadequately immunized pregnant women because this affords protection against neonatal tetanus
  **E.** Immune globulins are considered safe

**272.** In scabies, transfer of parasites is by direct skin-to-skin contact; infection can also occur during sexual contact. Which of the following is currently considered the treatment of choice for scabies?
  **A.** Lindane 1% shampoo
  **B.** Crotamiton 10% cream
  **C.** Topical sulfur ointment
  **D.** Permethrin 1% shampoo
  **E.** Permethrin 5% cream

**273.** Infants with macrocephaly, hydrocephalus, mental retardation, and chorioretinitis are most likely to have congenital
  **A.** coccidioidomycosis
  **B.** cysticercosis
  **C.** dermatophytosis
  **D.** toxoplasmosis
  **E.** rubella syndrome

**274.** Concerning the epidemiology of histoplasmosis, which of the following is **INCORRECT**?
  **A.** There is a high prevalence of the infection in the Mississippi and Ohio River Valleys
  **B.** Soil or dust is the source of primary infection
  **C.** Transmission is by inhalation of airborne spores
  **D.** It can be directly transmitted from person to person
  **E.** No vaccine is currently available

**275.** Concerning genital herpes simplex virus infection, which of the following is true?

**A.** It is a disease that may be chronic and recurring and for which no known cure exists

**B.** Systemic acyclovir treatment can eradicate the infection

**C.** Treatment with systemic acyclovir decreases the subsequent risk, frequency, and severity of recurrences, even after the drug is discontinued

**D.** Topical therapy with acyclovir is therapeutically equivalent to oral therapy with the drug

**E.** Transmission occurs only at the time of open lesions

**276.** Regarding nosocomial infections, all of the following are true **EXCEPT**

**A.** with improved control methods, nosocomial infections currently occur at a ratio of only 1% to 2% of US hospital admissions

**B.** referral hospitals generally have higher rates than community hospitals

**C.** urinary tract infections are the most common hospital-acquired infections

**D.** the mortality rate for nosocomial bacteremia is higher than for community-acquired bacteremia

**E.** gram-positive organisms are the most common causes of nosocomial bloodstream infection

**277.** Students in a junior high school became ill with symptoms of headache, chills, nausea, and vomiting. Investigation showed that the illness was confined to students who attended the 9:30 to 11:15 home economics classes on that day, where fruit punch and cookies prepared the previous evening were served. The incubation period ranged from 5 minutes to 2 hours. The punch was stored overnight in three 5-gal water containers with galvanized metal linings. The punch was transferred to plastic pitchers immediately before it was served. Which of the following is **CORRECT?**
**A.** The short incubation period suggests staphylococcal food poisoning
**B.** Food poisoning is unlikely here because of the absence of diarrhea and the foods involved in this case (punch and cookies)
**C.** The incubation period and the storage of the punch suggests *Clostridium perfringens* as the etiologic agent
**D.** The short incubation period and the storage of the punch suggest chemical food poisoning
**E.** Culture of the remaining punch would probably help in the diagnosis

**278.** Vaccines that are routinely administered to children in the United States include all of the following **EXCEPT**
**A.** diphtheria
**B.** tetanus
**C.** pertussis
**D.** influenza
**E.** *Haemophilus influenzae* type B

**279.** Other vaccines routinely administered to children in the United States include all of the following **EXCEPT**
**A.** measles
**B.** pneumococcus
**C.** rubella
**D.** polio
**E.** mumps

**280.** Which of the following is **LEAST** likely to be true? A person who is infected with HIV
**A.** may be asymptomatic
**B.** may have been infected by heterosexual contacts with infected partners

    **C.** may have been infected by daily nonsexual household contact with an infected family member
    **D.** may be a transfusion patient
    **E.** may be a child born to an infected mother

**281.** Which of the following is true concerning giardiasis?
    **A.** Transmission occurs by inhalation of infected droplets
    **B.** Stool smears usually show an abundance of leukocytes
    **C.** Diarrhea is typically greasy and foul-smelling
    **D.** Waterborne transmission does not occur if the municipal water supply is chlorinated
    **E.** Water that has been frozen and free of subsequent contamination is safe

**282.** All of the following are true concerning hepatitis B and the delta virus **EXCEPT**
    **A.** combined hepatitis B virus and delta virus infection is recognized to cause hepatitis outbreaks with unusually high mortality in parenteral drug abusers
    **B.** delta superinfection of hepatitis B virus carriers frequently causes transformation from no or mild chronic liver disease to severe, progressive chronic active hepatitis
    **C.** in the United States, infection with delta virus has been observed among persons with frequent blood (and blood product) exposures
    **D.** in the United States, most cases of acute hepatitis B infection and hepatitis D are associated with blood transfusions or with needle-stick injuries in health care workers
    **E.** hepatitis B vaccine has significantly decreased the incidence of hepatitis D among health care workers

**283.** Acquired immunodeficiency syndrome (AIDS) has been recognized in infants as a result of transmission of human immunodeficiency virus (HIV) from infected mothers before, at, or shortly after birth. Estimates of the rate of HIV transmission to such infants (from their infected mothers) in the absence of zidovudine prophylaxis range from approximately
    **A.** 1% to 4%
    **B.** 5% to 14%
    **C.** 15% to 19%
    **D.** 20% to 40%
    **E.** more than 40%

**Questions 284–286:**
Match the following diseases with their description.

    **A.** trichomoniasis
    **B.** lymphogranuloma venereum
    **C.** chancroid
    **D.** gonorrhea
    **E.** syphilis

**284.** A chronic and progressive bacterial disease of the skin and mucous membranes of the external genitalia, inguinal, and anal regions with low communicability. Laboratory diagnosis is based on demonstration of intracytoplasmic rod-shaped organisms in Giemsa-stained smears of granulation tissue or biopsy specimens.

**285.** This chlamydial disease is found more commonly in the tropical regions of the world. It is characterized by a swelling of lymph glands in the inguinal region, frequently accompanied by genital swelling. It can be diagnosed by complement fixation or by specific micro-IF test.

**286.** Worldwide, it is one of the most common of the sexually transmitted diseases and continues to be a frequent cause of blindness.

**Questions 287–291:**
Match the following diseases with their description.

    **A.** chancroid
    **B.** lymphogranuloma venereum
    **C.** condyloma acuminata
    **D.** trichomoniasis
    **E.** bacterial vaginosis (*Gardnerella*-associated vaginitis)

**287.** Causes nonirritating, malodorous, thin, gray discharge and, microscopically, "clue cells"

**288.** Recommended therapeutic regimen is 2 g metronidazole by mouth in a single dose

**289.** Cryotherapy and podophyllin are treatment options

**290.** Diagnosis is best made by isolation of *Haemophilus ducreyi* from ulcers or fluctuant nodes

**291.** Drug regimen of choice: doxycycline 100 mg PO b.i.d. for 21 days

**Questions 292–295:**
Match the following diseases with their description.

    **A.** rabies
    **B.** tetanus
    **C.** rat-bite fever
    **D.** leptospirosis
    **E.** lymphocytic choriomeningitis

**292.** Distributed worldwide, it has an incubation period of 3 to 21 days; case fatality rate varies from 30% to 90%. Laboratory tests are of little help in diagnosis. Reservoir: intestines of humans and animals.

**293.** Incubation period in humans is as short as 10 days and up to 1 year; rapidly fatal paralytic infection; incidence uniform throughout the year. Rare airborne spread. All warm-blooded mammals are susceptible. Natural immunity in humans is not known.

**294.** Sudden onset with chills, fever, prostration, and myalgia; evidence of renal involvement often present; fatality rate up to 20% in cases with jaundice and renal damage.

**295.** An endemic viral infection of animals, transmissible to humans; deaths are rare; organism is transferred from house mouse to human in feces and urine; nature of illness established by virus isolation.

**Questions 296–300:**
Match each type of food poisoning with the most appropriate attribute.
Each may be used once, more than once, or not at all.

- **A.** short incubation period
- **B.** incubation period of 15 to 50 days
- **C.** identified by isolation of organisms in stools of affected individuals and in implicated food
- **D.** found in certain species of mushrooms
- **E.** caused by ingestion of raw marine fish

**296.** *Clostridium perfringens*

**297.** Outbreaks of chemical etiology

**298.** Staphylococcus

**299.** Amanita toxin

**300.** Hepatitis A

**Questions 301–305:**
Select the most pertinent feature of food- or water-borne disease outbreaks caused by each etiology. Each may be used once, more than once, or not at all.

- **A.** outbreaks related to home-preserved vegetables
- **B.** outbreaks usually involve beef
- **C.** outbreaks related to ingestion of coral reef fish, raw or cooked
- **D.** isolation of organism from epidemiologically implicated food or ill patient's stools
- **E.** patients may have eosinophilia and periorbital edema

**301.** Salmonella

**302.** *Trichinella spiralis*

**303.** *Clostridium perfringens*

**304.** *C. botulinum*

**305.** Ciguatera

**Questions 306 and 307:**
Which disease's epidemiology is best described in each question?

- **A.** anthrax
- **B.** plague
- **C.** tetanus
- **D.** brucellosis
- **E.** tularemia

**306.** Spore remains viable in soil for many years. More of a problem in animals than humans; disease rarely spreads from person to person.

**307.** Transmission to humans by ingestion of raw milk and direct contact with infected animal or its body parts; strong rural concentration of the disease. Men are more frequently infected, and the disease is not transmitted from person to person.

**308.** Regarding streptococcal disease, which of the following is **INCORRECT**?
- **A.** Anal, vaginal, and pharyngeal carriers have all been responsible for nosocomial outbreaks of wound infections
- **B.** Epidemics of puerperal fever may occur in institutions where aseptic techniques are faulty
- **C.** In epidemics following surgical procedures, if an operating room person is identified as a carrier, eradication of the infection is usually easily accomplished with one course of antibiotics
- **D.** Acute glomerulonephritis is a documented complication of streptococcal skin infection
- **E.** Rheumatic heart disease has decreased significantly as a result of improved treatment options

**309.** All of the following are components of the proper definition of a nosocomial infection **EXCEPT**
- **A.** infection originates in a hospital or other health care facility
- **B.** the infection was not present or incubating at the time of admission
- **C.** includes infections acquired in the hospital but appearing after discharge
- **D.** the infection may have been acquired from another patient
- **E.** the infection would not have come from a hospital employee

**310.** Which of the following is the single most important element in any hospital infection control program?
  **A.** Judicious use of new broad-spectrum antibiotics (eg, third generation cephalosporins)
  **B.** Hand washing
  **C.** Use of gloves
  **D.** Placing appropriate patients in isolation
  **E.** Use of masks and gowns

**311.** Which of the following is **INCORRECT** concerning perinatal hepatitis B virus (HBV) exposure in the United States?
  **A.** All pregnant women should be routinely tested for hepatitis B surface antigen (HBsAg) during an early prenatal visit in each pregnancy
  **B.** Infants born to HBsAg-positive mothers should receive hepatitis B immune globulin (HBIg) intramuscularly, preferably within 12 hours of birth
  **C.** Infants born to HBsAg-positive mothers should receive a series of hepatitis B vaccine beginning 3 months after a dose of HBIg
  **D.** HBIg and hepatitis B vaccination do not interfere with routine childhood immunizations
  **E.** HBsAg-positive mothers may breast-feed, if the infants have begun prophylaxis

**312.** Identify the **CORRECT** statement regarding paralytic shellfish poisoning.
  **A.** Can be prevented by adequate cooking and storage of the shellfish
  **B.** Usually follows the ingestion of lobsters and crabs
  **C.** Mainstay of therapy is supportive measures but may be fatal in previously healthy people
  **D.** Outbreaks occur year round without seasonal peaks
  **E.** Incubation period is 12 to 24 hours

**313.** Regarding primary amebic meningoencephalitis (PEM), identify the **INCORRECT** statement.
  **A.** It is caused by free-living amebae of genus *Naegleria* and *Acanthamoeba*
  **B.** It is transmitted by exposure of nasal passages to contaminated water or through open skin lesions

**C.** It occurs mainly in active young people of both sexes
**D.** Adequate treatment is usually successful
**E.** The typical syndrome includes meningoencephalitis with sore throat, headache, nausea, vomiting, fever, and death within 10 days

**314.** Concerning rabies incidence, prevention, and treatment in the United States, identify the **INCORRECT** statement.
   **A.** The postexposure prophylaxis schedule recommended by the Centers for Disease Control and Prevention for those not previously vaccinated includes one dose of Human Rabies Immune Globulin (HRIG) and five doses of Human Diploid Cell Rabies Vaccine (HDCV) over a 28-day period
   **B.** Preexposure vaccination should be offered to persons in high-risk groups and consists of three doses of HDCV
   **C.** Postexposure prophylaxis combining local wound treatment, vaccination, and passive immunization is uniformly effective if appropriately used
   **D.** Rabies in humans has increased in the United States since 1950
   **E.** Wild animals now constitute the largest potential source of infection for both humans and domestic animals in the United States

**315.** In a common-source outbreak of salmonellosis, the mean incubation period would most likely be about
   **A.** 1 hour
   **B.** 4 hours
   **C.** 24 hours
   **D.** 4 days
   **E.** 1 week

**316.** Which of the following foods is most conducive to *Salmonella* growth?
   **A.** Sliced bread
   **B.** Pickled pigs' feet
   **C.** Turkey
   **D.** Celery
   **E.** Carbonated beverages

317. Identify the **INCORRECT** statement regarding *Salmonella* infections.
    A. Foods containing a single *Salmonella*-contaminated egg can cause outbreaks of severe illness
    B. Fruits and vegetables have never been reported to be vehicles for *Salmonella* infections
    C. *Salmonella* outbreaks associated with eggs should be reported to the state agriculture department and the US Department of Agriculture
    D. When ingested in sufficient quantity, *Salmonella* infections can be fatal in an otherwise healthy host
    E. Standard cooking methods for many egg-containing foods, such as Hollandaise sauce, meringue, and soft-boiled eggs, may not kill *Salmonella*

318. Concerning the use of amantadine in the prevention of influenza, which of the following statements is true?
    A. It is now fairly well established that the antiviral drug amantadine hydrochloride is ineffective in preventing illness caused by influenza type A viruses
    B. Amantadine is effective against influenza type B viruses
    C. Amantadine is likely to cause troublesome side effects in younger adults and therefore it is indicated only for individuals 65 or older
    D. To be fully effective as prophylaxis, amantadine must be taken once a week for the duration of influenza activity in the community
    E. In high-risk individuals vaccinated during an outbreak of influenza A, it is appropriate to use amantadine 2 weeks after vaccination while antibodies are being developed

319. Regarding bubonic plague, all of the following are true **EXCEPT**
    A. the incubation period is 2 to 6 days
    B. plague is clinically characterized in humans by lymphadenitis and septicemia
    C. the plague bacillus is *Yersinia pestis*
    D. the disease is transmitted by tick bites
    E. it occurs largely in the western third of the United States

**320.** Which is **CORRECT** concerning prevention and treatment of plague?
   **A.** There is no specific treatment
   **B.** Streptomycin and tetracyclines are effective
   **C.** Sulfadiazine is the drug of choice
   **D.** There is no immunizing agent
   **E.** Prophylactic use of antibiotics is not effective

**321.** Which is **INCORRECT** regarding the transmission of pertussis?
   **A.** It is most communicable during catarrhal and before paroxysmal stage
   **B.** The infective agent is carried in secretions from the respiratory tract
   **C.** Transmission is airborne, probably by droplets
   **D.** Domestic animal carriers provide a reservoir
   **E.** Incubation period is commonly 7 to 10 days

**322.** Which is **CORRECT** concerning the treatment of diphtheria?
   **A.** Antibiotics are a satisfactory substitute for antitoxin
   **B.** Both antitoxin and penicillin are indicated
   **C.** Erythromycin is not an effective substitute for penicillin
   **D.** Antitoxin should be administered only after receiving bacteriologic confirmation of the diagnosis
   **E.** Carrier states require no treatment

**323.** The gastrointestinal tract is a portal of entry for
   **A.** coccidioidomycosis
   **B.** onchocerciasis
   **C.** dengue fever
   **D.** brucellosis
   **E.** leishmaniasis

**324.** Regarding tuberculin skin testing, which is **INCORRECT?**
   - **A.** The Mantoux test, not the multiple puncture test, is the preferred method of identifying persons infected with *Mycobacterium tuberculosis*
   - **B.** A reaction of 5 mm is now considered significant for persons with known HIV infection or those who are close contacts of infectious cases of tuberculosis (TB)
   - **C.** Screening for TB can identify infected persons at high risk of clinical disease who would benefit from therapy
   - **D.** Absence of a reaction does not exclude the diagnosis of TB
   - **E.** History of vaccination with BCG invalidates the standard guidelines for the interpretation of the TB skin test

**325.** After receipt of recombinant DNA hepatitis B vaccine, which of the following represents an immune response?
   - **A.** HBsAg
   - **B.** Anti-HBs
   - **C.** HBcAg
   - **D.** IgM anti-HBc
   - **E.** All indicate an immune response to the vaccine

# Communicable Diseases

## Answers and Discussion

**75. (B)** Enterotoxigenic *Escherichia coli (E. coli)* is the most likely pathogen. It is the most common cause of diarrhea in travelers. The diarrhea is usually characterized by watery consistency and abdominal cramping. Vomiting and high temperatures are unusual. Diarrhea usually lasts 5 days and is usually self-limited. **(Ref. 2, p. 62; Ref. 22, pp. 531–533)**

**76. (A)** Prophylaxis with trimethoprim-sulfamethoxazole can prevent this diarrhea. However, this illness is usually self-limited and requires only hydration and rest. The problem associated with widespread use of antibiotic prophylaxis is that it can lead to resistance. Pepto-Bismol has been shown to lessen the duration and severity of diarrhea associated with *Escherichia coli.* **(Ref. 2, p. 62)**

**77. (E)** When traveling to countries where the water is unsafe, it is necessary to carry one's own water or only use water that has been purified for drinking. Chlorine tablets can be taken on such trips to accomplish this purpose. Water can also be purified by adding two to four drops of 5% chlorine bleach or by adding five to ten drops of 2% tincture of iodine per quart. Boiling water is an even better purifying method. It is best to avoid fruits washed in local untreated water; however, consumption of fruit after removing an intact peeling is safer. **(Ref. 2, pp. 62, 179)**

**78. (A)** Yellow fever vaccination is required for travel to tropical Africa and Central and South America. This vaccination provides protection for 10 years. Vaccination for smallpox is no longer necessary as it has been eradicated. The last case was seen in October 1977. Meningococcal vaccination is *recommended* during the seasons it is most likely to be transmitted in those areas where transmission is possible (Saudi Arabia, Nepal, etc). Japanese encephalitis is *recommended* for travel to high risk areas in rural Asia. The typhoid vaccine is *recommended* for travel to endemic areas. **(Ref. 2,** pp. 60–61)

**79. (B)** Hemorrhagic colitis has been associated with the *E. coli* strain 0157:H7. Hemolytic uremic syndrome has been associated with *Shigella dysenteriae* and *Salmonella typhi.* Disseminated *Yersinia* infection and salmonellosis can be associated with meningitis and osteomyelitis. Acute reactive arthritis has been associated with *Shigella, Salmonella, Yersinia,* and *Campylobacter* infections. **(Ref. 22,** pp. 531, 667, 668, 675–677)

**80. (D)** In general, pregnant travelers should avoid live vaccines. Included among the live vaccines are measles, mumps, and rubella (MMR); yellow fever; oral polio vaccine (OPV); and oral typhoid. The MMR is an absolute contraindication during pregnancy. The injectable form of the polio vaccine (IPV) is the preferred vaccine against polio during pregnancy. However, if immediate protection is needed, the oral vaccine is permissible. Injectable typhoid is permitted if the risk justifies it. Vaccinating the mother against tetanus also affords protection to the unborn fetus. It is preferred to delay vaccination until the second or third trimester. As an aside, hepatitis B vaccine can also be administered to a pregnant patient. **(Ref. 71,** p. 76; **Ref. 17,** pp. 19–23)

**81. (B)** In general for HIV patients and other immunocompromised patients, the live vaccines are to be avoided. However, in the case of measles, mumps, and rubella (MMR), it is thought that the benefits outweigh the risks because measles can be so devastating in these patients. BCG should not be given to immunocompromised patients. **(Ref. 2,** p. 68)

**82. (C)** The measles, mumps, and rubella (MMR) vaccine is not appropriate for the 6-month visit but rather is given after 12 to 15 months. Prior to this time the infant is protected by maternal antibodies (passive immunity), and the vaccine would be inactivated. (**Ref. 68,** pp. 43, 44)

83. **(A)** Typhoid can be common among young children, but they usually have mild cases. The importance of vaccination increases as access to reasonable medical care decreases. The injectable form of the typhoid vaccine is preferred for HIV-positive persons. (**Ref. 68,** pp. 105–111)

84. **(D)** Immune globulin can be given either 2 weeks after measles or MMR immunization or 6 weeks (preferably 3 months) before measles, mumps, rubella (MMR) immunization. Immune globulin should be given with caution to persons with an allergy or sensitivity to mercury or thimerosal. Intramuscular injections should be avoided when possible in patients with coagulation disorders, platelet defects, or thrombocytopenia. Immune globulin can be given with yellow fever and oral polio vaccines (OPV). (**Ref. 68,** pp. 83–85)

85. **(A)** Measles vaccine (usually as MMR) is not contraindicated for HIV-positive persons. It is felt that the disease manifestations of measles in these persons far outweigh the risks of vaccination. However, measles vaccination is contraindicated in persons with AIDS. In people with congenital immunodeficiency, the MMR is contraindicated. Persons born prior to 1957 probably have natural immunity from previous infection. The MMR is always contraindicated in pregnancy. (**Ref. 68,** pp. 42–47)

86. **(C)** Measles is more common in children but not more severe. The risk of complications are highest among the very young or the very old. The incubation period for measles is 10 to 12 days. Usually the first symptoms are fever and malaise, followed by cough, coryza, and conjunctivitis. Prompt administration of immune globulin to exposed individuals can alter clinical disease. (**Ref. 22,** pp. 825, 826)

87. **(C)** Many of the mentioned strategies are useful; however, the most successful has been the routine immunization of children through the enactment and enforcement of school immunization laws. Passive immunity is associated with the newborn period

until about 12 months of age and is conferred by maternal antibodies. (**Ref. 2,** pp. 65–68)

**88.** **(C)** The World Health Organization makes yearly recommendations to the Centers for Disease Control and Prevention. It is necessary to do so this often because of the changing strains. Influenza A epidemics are more common than B epidemics, hence the two A strains and one B strain. Guillain-Barré syndrome has not been observed in association with influenza vaccines since 1976. The influenza vaccine should be given annually to high risk groups during the fall season. This reduces their risk substantially if the circulating strain is antigenically similar to the vaccine. (**Ref. 2,** p. 84)

**89.** **(C)** Efforts to control influenza mortality in the United States have been most successful with two methods: immunization and chemoprophylaxis with amantidine. Immunization of high risk groups is still the mainstay for influenza mortality control. (**Ref. 2,** p. 84)

**90.** **(D)** Varicella has been known to spread by all of the routes mentioned; however, blood-borne is the least common method. (**Ref. 2,** p. 91)

**91.** **(A)** Chemoprophylaxis with rifampin is given to all household contacts in families with children under 4 years of age in contact with a patient with *Haemophilus influenzae* infection. Both a three-stage and a two-stage vaccination with subsequent boosters are available. Immunization against *H. influenzae* usually begins at the 2-month visit in a normal healthy infant. Aggressive treatment with chloramphenicol and ampicillin is preferable in the case of life-threatening illnesses (eg, meningitis, epiglottiditis). (**Ref. 2,** pp. 86, 87)

**92.** **(B)** Ninety-five percent of *Haemophilus influenzae* meningitis cases occur in children under 5 years of age. Peak incidence is in children 6 to 7 months old. The incidence is lowest in the summer and peaks in the fall and spring. The incidence of *H. influenzae* infection is three times higher in the black population than the white population. The incidence of infection with *H. influenzae* has increased in the past few decades. (**Ref. 2,** p. 86)

**93. (D)** *Streptococcus pneumoniae* is the most common cause of community-acquired bacterial pneumonia. It is also responsible for most cases of otitis media. Pnemococcus, *Neisseria,* and *Haemophilus* are the most common causes of meningitis. The case fatality rate for meningitis secondary to pneumococcus is high in persons over 40 years of age. Lung abscess is a rare complication of pneumococcal infection. Pneumovax is recommended for older persons. **(Ref. 2,** p. 87)

**94. (C)** The "3-day measles" or rubella is characterized by a relatively mild maculopapular rash that lasts 3 days or less. The rash begins on the face and spreads downward. Contraction of rubella during the first trimester is particularly dangerous and may result in numerous congenital abnormalities of the fetus. Possible cardiac manifestations included are patent ductus arteriosus, pulmonary stenosis, and myocardial necrosis. **(Ref. 2,** pp. 70, 71)

**95. (B)** Precocious puberty has been associated with congenital rubella infection as has diabetes mellitus, growth retardation, and growth hormone deficiency. **(Ref. 2,** p. 71)

**96. (C)** The most effective strategy for the prevention and control of pertussis is active immunization. This highly contagious infection has a secondary attack rate of close to 90%. Antibiotics can eliminate infection and if given early enough (in the catarrhal phase) can ameliorate symptoms. **(Ref. 2,** p. 75; **Ref. 7,** p. 660)

**97. (B)** Pneumonia is the most common cause of mortality in adults. Sepsis and encephalitis are also common causes of mortality in children. **(Ref. 2,** p. 90)

**98. (C)** Bacille Calmette-Guérin (BCG) vaccine is absolutely contraindicated for patients with HIV. Measles, mumps, rubella is preferred to risking measles infection. Pneumococcal and tetanus vaccines are also permissible. Inactivated polio vaccine and injectable typhoid vaccine do not contain live organisms; therefore these are also appropriate for HIV-positive persons. **(Ref. 26)**

**99. (D)** Immune globulin is appropriate for HIV-positive travelers. The injectable form of the polio vaccine and the injectable typhoid vaccine are preferable to the live, oral forms. Yellow fever vaccination is also not recommended except in the case of substantial risk in an HIV-positive patient. The bacille Calmette-Guérin vaccine is never indicated for HIV-positive patients. (**Ref. 67, pp.** 129, 130)

**100.** (**B**)  Rubella vaccine virus is the only one to be isolated from breast milk. However, this should not be considered a contraindication for immunization in the postnatal period. There has been no indication that babies receiving breast milk from mothers immunized against rubella have been harmed. (**Ref. 46**)

**101.** (**A**)  Breast feeding, diarrhea, low-grade fever, and prematurity are not contraindications to receiving the oral polio vaccine. However, persons with household contacts who are immunocompromised should not receive the oral polio vaccine. (**Ref. 68, pp.** 139, 140)

**102.** (**C**)  A significantly elevated temperature should be considered a precaution when considering diphtheria-pertussis-tetanus (DPT) vaccination. A family history of convulsions, sudden infant death syndrome, diarrhea, or prematurity should not be considered a precaution to administering the DPT vaccine. (**Ref. 68, pp.** 139, 140)

**103.** (**C**)  Barrier methods and total abstinence from sexual activity are the major modes of primary prevention. Contact tracing and subsequent treatment also contribute to primary prevention. Screening programs have their best efficacy in high-risk populations only. (**Ref. 2, pp.** 108, 109)

**104.** (**B**)  Syphilis in all its stages is curable even today with penicillin. Treatment of syphilis may reduce possible concurrent transmission of other sexually transmitted diseases (eg, HIV). During the last half of the 1980s, the incidence of primary and secondary syphilis increased dramatically. This was reflected most strongly in the low income, minority, heterosexual populations, but not among homosexuals. (**Ref. 2, pp.** 102, 103)

**105.** (**A**)  There was an overall decrease in the incidence of gonorrhea in the US population from 1975 to 1989 of approximately 30%. This decrease was thought to be secondary to a reduction in high-risk sexual practices of white Americans. Unfortunately, this message is not reaching the inner-city, teenager and adolescent minority population, as transmission rates in this group are increasing. (**Ref. 2,** p. 104)

**106.** (**C**)  In 1976, clinically significant PPNG became evident. The three classes of drugs now less effective are tetracyclines, penicillins, and aminoglycosides (especially spectinomycin). The recommendations for treatment of gonococcal infections tend now toward third-generation cephalosporins. (**Ref. 2,** p. 104)

**107.** (**B**)  *Chlamydia trachomatis* is the cause of the most common sexually transmitted bacterial genital infection. (**Ref. 2,** p. 104)

**108.** (**A**)  Plasmid-mediated resistance has increasingly become a problem with gonococcal therapy with tetracyclines. (**Ref. 2,** p. 104)

**109.** (**A**)  Chromosomally mediated resistance has contributed to treatment failure of gonococcal infections with penicillins and tetracyclines. (**Ref. 2,** p. 104)

**110.** (**B**)  The cause of initial onset of multiple painful genital lesions of a sexually transmitted origin is most likely herpes simplex, type 2. (**Ref. 2,** p. 105)

**111.** (**B**)  Viral isolation of HSV-2 from tissue culture is the definitive method for identification of this viral infection. The yield is further increased if this is a primary infection and when the lesions are vesicular (as opposed to ulcerative). Presumptive diagnosis can be made from the Tzanck preparation in the office setting. Darkfield examination technique establishes the definitive diagnosis of *Treponema pallidum* infection. Fluorescent monoclonal antibody stain helps establish the diagnosis of *Chlamydia trachomatis*. (**Ref. 2,** p. 111)

**112.** (**C**)  Squamous cell carcinoma of the cervix has been strongly associated with HSV-2 infection. Anal, vaginal, and vulvar carcinoma have been linked to human papilloma virus. Hepatocellular carcinoma has been associated with hepatitis B virus. (**Ref. 2,** p. 108)

**113.** (**B**)  Aseptic meningitis has been associated with HSV-2 infection. Epididymitis has been associated with *Neisseria gonor-*

*rhoeae* and *Chlamydia trachomatis.* Penile carcinoma has been linked to human papilloma virus. Prostatitis may be linked to *N. gonorrhoeae.* Vulvovaginitis has been associated with candidal infection. (**Ref. 2,** p. 100)

114. **(B)** Acyclovir is still the treatment of choice to reduce morbidity and possible recurrences of HSV-2 clinical manifestations. (**Ref. 2,** p. 112)

115. **(B)** In those patients having HSV-2 antibodies, only one in three ever noticed having symptoms related to HSV-2 infection. And in those patients with primary HSV-2, 75% of their sexual contacts never noticed any genital lesions. HSV-2 is the leading cause of genital ulceration in the United States. The incidence of neonatal herpes has increased as a direct consequence of an increase in genital herpes lesions. (**Ref. 2,** pp. 105, 106)

116. **(B)** HPV cannot yet be determined by viral culture. Detection of koilocytes on cytologic smears, morphologic features on colposcopy, immunochemical stains, or nucleic acid sequences are the methods most often used. A fourth method includes determination of HPV infection from cervical smears by using polymerase chain reactions (PCR). With the aid of this technique, HPV is being detected despite an otherwise normal Papanicolaou smear. (**Ref. 2,** pp. 106, 107)

117. **(B)** HPV can be transmitted in the absence of genital lesions or symptoms and probably occurs mostly under these circumstances. If appropriate follow-up is not done after a suspicious Papanicolaou smear, there could be progression to cervical carcinoma and possible death. (**Ref. 2,** pp. 106, 107)

118. **(A)** The US vaccination program for the hepatitis B virus (HBV) has traditionally focused on the vaccination of health care workers, institutionalized patients, and hemodialysis patients. However, these persons are not responsible for the majority of known HBV infection transmissions. Most cases are transmitted through sexual contact or intravenous drug use. Vaccination of persons who handle food should more likely include hepatitis A virus (HAV) vaccine, since transmission of this type is fecal-oral. (**Ref. 2,** p. 107)

**119.** (E) Possible long-term effects associated with hepatitis B infection include chronic carrier status, fulminant hepatitis, chronic active hepatitis and hepatocellular carcinoma. (**Ref. 2,** p. 107)

**120.** (B) Gonococcal infection during pregnancy has been associated with an increased risk of premature rupture of membranes, chorioamnionitis, low birth weight, and prematurity. Spontaneous abortion is also a possible outcome; however, this is mostly associated with primary herpes infection. (**Ref. 2,** p. 108)

**121.** (D) Concentrating on promoting safer sexual practices for high-risk groups is currently the most cost-effective. Cesarean delivery and prenatal screening are not currently considered to be cost-effective. Reducing the duration of infectivity is not considered to be reliable at this time. (**Ref. 2,** pp. 108, 109)

**122.** (B) Human papilloma virus (HPV) has been associated with several neoplasms including vulvar, vaginal, anal, and cervical. Testicular cancer is not associated with HPV infection. (**Ref. 2,** p. 101)

**123.** (A) Penile cancer has been strongly associated with human papilloma virus. (**Ref. 2,** p. 101)

**124.** (B) Hepatocellular carcinoma has been strongly associated with hepatitis B infection. (**Ref. 2,** p. 101)

**125.** (C) Non-Hodgkin's lymphoma has been linked to human immunodeficiency virus infection. (**Ref. 2,** p. 101)

**126.** (A) Human papilloma virus has been strongly associated with anal carcinoma. (**Ref. 2,** p. 101)

**127.** (B) *Chlamydia trachomatis* is the most likely sexually transmitted disease associated with the triad of urethritis, conjunctivitis, and arthritis. This syndrome is called Reiter's syndrome. (**Ref. 2,** p. 100)

**128.** (A) The treatment of choice for *Chlamydia trachomatis* is doxycycline. Tetracycline is also an alternative. Metronidazole is the treatment of choice for *Gardnerella vaginalis*. Penicillin is still the treatment for syphilis. Cephalosporins are becoming significant therapy for gonococcal infections. (**Ref. 2,** p. 112)

**129. (A)** Treatment for Reiter's syndrome is directed toward relief of symptoms. Nonsteroidal anti-inflammatories and analgesics are used as with rheumatoid arthritis for inflammation and pain relief. Use of antibiotics is unclear. However, systemic steroids are not used with Reiter's syndrome because of fear that this will aggravate the dermatologic manifestations of the syndrome (eg, keratoderma, blenorrhagia, and mucosal lesions). **(Ref. 22,** pp. 764, 765)

**130. (C)** Both gonococcal arthritis and Reiter's syndrome are likely to be characterized by the presence of conjunctivitis. **(Ref. 22,** p. 556)

**131. (A)** Reiter's syndrome is most likely to be associated with the presence of balanitis. **(Ref. 22,** p. 556)

**132. (B)** Gonococcal arthritis is most likely to affect the upper extremities, whereas Reiter's syndrome is most likely to affect the lower extremeties. **(Ref. 22,** p. 1689)

**133. (B)** Gonococcal arthritis responds to treatment with penicillin, whereas Reiter's syndrome is unresponsive to penicillin. **(Ref. 22,** p. 1689)

**134. (B)** AIDS is most frequently reported following an opportunistic infection. The opportunistic infection that occurs earliest is the AIDS-defining illness. The most frequently reported AIDS-defining illness is *Pneumocystis carinii* pneumonia. Kaposi's sarcoma has mostly been associated with young homosexual males. **(Ref. 2,** p. 117; **Ref. 28)**

**135. (A)** A survey of seroprevalence in the New York area in 1985 revealed a seropositive rate of approximately 57% in intravenous drug users. However, the seropositive rate in childbearing women was 14%. This latter group is thought to represent heterosexual transmission. **(Ref. 2,** p. 119)

**136. (B)** In parts of Southeast Asia, the incidence of AIDS among prostitutes is high. Safer sexual practices would be the most advantageous method to try to control the spread of HIV infection in that region. **(Ref. 2,** p. 119)

**137. (B)** Although unintentional injuries, prematurity, and cancer are very common causes of years of potential life lost, HIV infection is the cause of years of potential life lost that is increasing the fastest. **(Ref. 2, p. 121)**

**138. (C)** Invasive cervical carcinoma, CD4-positive T-lymphocyte count <200/mm$^3$ or CD4-positive T-lymphocyte percentage of total lymphocytes <14, pulmonary tuberculosis, and recurrent pneumonia are all part of the revised classification system for HIV infection and expanded case definition for AIDS surveillance. Recurrent yeast infections may be an indication of HIV seropositivity in women; however, it is not a part of the expanded case definition. **(Ref. 28)**

**139. (E)** Squamous cell carcinoma of the anus has been associated with male homosexuality but not necessarily with HIV infection. Kaposi's sarcoma, non-Hodgkin's lymphoma, and invasive cervical carcinoma are neoplastic conditions that have been associated with HIV infection. **(Ref. 2, p. 108)**

**140. (A)** In 1993 the greatest risk factor associated with heterosexual HIV transmission was, of course, having a partner who was HIV-positive. The second most common risk factor was being the sexual partner of an intravenous drug user. **(Ref. 29)**

**141. (D)** Common symptoms include fever, malaise, chills, vomiting, headaches, and joint pain. Diarrhea is uncommon. **(Ref. 2, pp. 173, 174)**

**142. (D)** Chloramphenicol is the drug of choice, but ampicillin, trimethoprim–sulfamethoxazole, and ciprofloxacin are all acceptable alternatives. **(Ref. 2, p. 175)**

**143. (C)** *Vibrio cholerae* is a gram-negative bacterium. Cholera symptoms are caused by a protein endotoxin that turns on the adenylate cyclase and increases electrolyte secretion into the intestinal lumen. Symptoms include rice-water stools and vomiting. It can be fatal in hours, and rehydration and electrolyte replacement is crucial. Water is the primary vehicle of infection. Bloody diarrhea is not usual with cholera. **(Ref. 2, pp. 176–178)**

**144. (D)** *Giardia lamblia* is a protozoan. (**Ref. 2**, pp. 186, 187)

**145. (C)** There is no evidence that *Legionella* is transmissible from person to person. (**Ref. 2**, pp. 181–183)

**146. (D)** The drug of choice for the treatment of *Giardia lamblia* is metronidazole. (**Ref. 2**, pp. 186–188)

**147. (D)** The cause of staphylococcal food poisoning is *Staphylococcus aureus*, which produces five heat-stable enterotoxins. Incubation period is 2 to 4 hours. Onset of nausea, vomiting, abdominal cramps, and salivation is abrupt. Staphylococci are found in low concentrations in contaminated food. (**Ref. 2**, pp. 194, 195)

**148. (A)** Salmonella is a gram-negative bacillus. Common signs and symptoms include diarrhea, abdominal cramps, fever, headaches, nausea, vomiting. Incubation is usually 6 to 48 hours. The source of contamination is usually raw meat and meat products, dairy products, and eggs. Prevention is by proper food handling, storage of food, and hand washing. (**Ref. 2**, pp. 195, 196)

**149. (D)** The drug of choice is chloramphenicol, whereas erythromycin is not effective. Patients with cholelithiasis often need cholecystectomy to eliminate carriage of *Salmonella typhi*. (**Ref. 2**, p. 195; **Ref. 74**, p. 263)

**150. (C)** *Clostridium perfringens* is an anaerobic gram-positive bacillus that is spore forming. It produces both heat-stable and heat-labile spores. Of the five toxicologic types, A and C cause human gastroenteritis. Common symptoms include abdominal cramps and diarrhea with occasional nausea. Fever and vomiting is usually absent. The incubation period is 6 to 24 hours. (**Ref. 2**, pp. 195, 196)

**151. (B)** *Clostridium botulinum* is a gram-positive anaerobic spore-forming bacillus. The spores are ubiquitous worldwide. Symptoms are caused by a preformed toxin. The toxin prevents the release of acetylcholine and interrupts the transmission of nerve impulses. The result is flaccid paralysis. The toxin is heat-labile, and 90% of outbreaks are due to home canning. (**Ref. 2**, pp. 196, 197)

**152. (C)** The incubation time is about 12 hours. **(Ref. 2, p. 198)**

**153. (E)** *Vibrio parahaemolyticus* is one of the leading causes of food-borne disease in Japan. Crustaceans from warm coastal marine waters are primarily affected. Ciguatera toxin is produced by dinoflagellates attached to algae on coral reefs. Fish eat the algae and concentrate the toxin. Paralytic shellfish poisoning is caused by ingestion of toxic dinoflagellates of the *Gonyaulax* species. Mollusks (mussels and clams) concentrate the neurotoxin saxitoxin. The toxic dinoflagellates bloom and cause "red tide." **(Ref. 2, p. 198)**

**154. (D)** Antidiarrheal agents are contraindicated because they prolong symptoms and increase the chance of bacteremia. **(Ref. 74, p. 263)**

**155. (D)** Urinary tract infections (UTIs) are the most common hospital acquired infections, accounting for about one third of all nosocomial infections. Surgical wound infections are the second most common, then lower respiratory tract infections, and lastly bloodstream infections. **(Ref. 2, pp. 203–205)**

**156. (D)** Gram-positive organisms including coagulase-negative staphylococci, *Staphylococcus aureus,* and the enterococci account for most nosocomial bloodstream infections. **(Ref. 2, p. 205)**

**157. (A)** *Legionella pneumophila* causes sporadic and occasionally epidemic lower respiratory tract infections in some hospitals. The organisms are spread through air conditioning units. **(Ref. 2, pp. 181, 182)**

**158. (C)** Chemotherapy, because of its immunosuppressive effects, predisposes individuals to a wide variety of infections. One of the most serious types is candidal bloodstream infections. These infections are associated with a significantly higher mortality rate compared to other bloodstream infections. **(Ref. 2, p. 205)**

**159. (D)** *Shigella* is easily transmitted by close person-to-person contact among children and by environmental contamination caused by children who are not toilet-trained. **(Ref. 2, p. 209)**

**160. (B)** Hepatitis A is spread by the fecal-oral route with transmission occurring between household and sexual contacts. Hepatitis A can also be spread through contact with contaminated fomites. It can survive on environmental surfaces for at least 1 month. Hepatitis A is typically a mild illness in young children but can cause substantial morbidity in adults. **(Ref. 2, p. 209)**

**161. (D)** Epidemic typhus has disappeared from much of the world except remote areas of Africa, Asia, and Central and South America. After an incubation period of 2 weeks, there is an abrupt onset of fever, chills, malaise, muscle aches, and severe headaches. Approximately 5 days later, a faint pink macular rash usually develops over the trunk. Tetracycline or chloramphenicol is usually curative if given early. Certain social factors that predispose to epidemic typhus, including overcrowding, poverty, and infrequent bathing or changing of clothes are especially common during cold weather or periods of war. **(Ref. 2, p. 233)**

**162. (A)** Scrub typhus, also known as tsutsugamushi disease, Japanese river fever, or tropical typhus, was first described in 16th-century China, and its ancient name means chigger fever. Most infections are of mild to moderate severity. Significant morbidity occurs regularly, however, and mortality rates range from 0 to 30% if untreated. Larval mites (chiggers) are the vectors and reservoirs. It is especially common in tropical and subtropical areas, including rain forests, riverbanks, and seashores. Doxycycline appears to be particularly reliable, and relapses are rare following its use. **(Ref. 2, p. 234)**

**163. (D)** Transmission to humans is through contamination of the bite wound or other skin breaks by vector feces. Most of the rickettsioses are characterized by the syndrome of severe headache, fever, myalgia, and rash of a specific pattern. There is no rash with Q fever. The rickettsiae are obligate intracellular parasites that can propagate only in living cells. Serology is the mainstay of laboratory diagnosis. Epidemic typhus, scrub and murine typhus, Brill-Zinsser disease, Q fever, and trench fever are all included in the human rickettsial diseases. Epidemic typhus is usually cured by tetracycline or chloramphenicol, and recovery is complete, with immunity to reinfection. However, the disease may recur decades later as Brill-Zinsser disease, which is usually milder with little or no rash. **(Ref. 2, pp. 231–235)**

**164. (C)** Q fever is essentially worldwide in distribution, although it is uncommon in the United States. After an incubation period of 2 to 4 weeks, fever, headache, malaise, weakness, and weight loss may last a few days or weeks, but no rash occurs. Domestic animals, including cattle, sheep, and goats are the main source of human illness. Location of dairy and other livestock operations away from population centers, disinfection, and appropriate disposal of infected animal tissues and regular spraying of cattle, sheep, and goats for control of ectoparasites may be effective. A formaldehyde vaccine is available commercially for epidemic typhus, but none is available for Q fever. (**Ref. 2,** p. 236)

**165. (B)** Q fever has no rash. (**Ref. 2,** pp. 235, 236)

**166. (A)** The natural life cycle of *Rochalimaea quintana* (trench fever) involves humans and the human body louse. (**Ref. 2,** pp. 235, 236)

**167. (C)** Rocky Mountain spotted fever and Q fever are important tick-borne typhus diseases. Rocky Mountain spotted fever has been recognized as a distinct entity in the United States and Canada since the late 1800s. (**Ref. 2,** pp. 235, 236)

**168. (B)** The classic form of *Yersinia pestis* infection in humans is bubonic plague. Other clinical forms (septicemia, pneumonic, meningeal) usually occur as complications of bubonic plague. In addition to flea bites, entry sites can include mucous membranes of the eye and oropharynx as well as broken skin. Within 2 to 7 days of exposure, onset of illness is heralded by fever, chills, pain in the area of lymph nodes, and eventually lymph node enlargement (bubo). It is best diagnosed by culture of material aspirated from a fluctuant bubo. The penicillins are not effective against *Y. pestis.* The most effective antibiotic is streptomycin. (**Ref. 2,** pp. 238, 239)

**169. (B)** Thirty minutes after malaria sporozoites are inoculated into a human, they enter hepatocytes, initiating the exoerythrocytic stage of development. Primary tissue schizogony of parasites takes 7 to 15 days in the liver. The schizonts then rupture, and the resulting merozoites enter RBCs. The RBC schizogenic cycle leads to maturation of the parasites, with ring-stage parasites becoming schizonts, which rupture and release merozoites into the bloodstream. These invade RBCs, and the erythrocytic cycle is continued. (**Ref. 2,** p. 240)

**170. (C)** The classic malarial illness occurs in a person with no prior exposure to the parasite, who experiences fever, chills, sweats, and headache, back pain, and malaise. Ideally the diagnosis of malaria in a febrile patient is confirmed by the identification of malaria parasites on a blood smear. **(Ref. 2,** p. 240)

**171. (A)** *P. falciparum* causes the most severe form of the disease, often with neurologic manifestations, renal failure, hemolytic anemia, hypoglycemia, and acute pulmonary edema. **(Ref. 2,** p. 240)

**172. (D)** Malaria in pregnancy is associated with low birth weight, anemia, acute pulmonary edema, still birth, premature labor, hypoglycemia, and fetal distress. **(Ref. 22,** p. 890)

**173. (B)** On the borders of Thailand, mefloquine resistance in *P. falciparum* has increased rapidly over the past 5 years. These regions contain the most drug-resistant parasites in the world and in the past have acted as harbingers of resistance patterns elsewhere in the tropics. The management of multidrug-resistant infections is difficult; quinine and tetracycline remain effective, but compliance with the 7-day regimen is poor. **(Ref. 66,** pp. 971–977)

**174. (B)** *Yersinia pestis* is the causative agent of the plague. It is maintained in natural reservoirs of infected rodents and fleas. The organism is a bipolar staining, gram-negative, nonsporulating, nonmotile coccobacillus. **(Ref. 2,** pp. 237–240)

**175. (A)** The causative agent of Q fever is *Coxiella burnetii.* Many infections are self-limited or mild, febrile illnesses. After an incubation period of 2 to 4 weeks, Q fever often manifests as fever, malaise, myalgia, headache, weakness, anorexia, and weight loss lasting several days to weeks. **(Ref. 2,** p. 232)

**176. (D)** *Rickettsia prowazekii* has been responsible for millions of cases of epidemic or louse typhus, causing uncounted deaths throughout history. The disease has disappeared from most of the world except remote areas of Africa, Asia, Central and South America. After an incubation period of 1 to 2 weeks, there is an abrupt onset of fever, chills, malaise, myalgia, severe headache, and macular rash. Mortality ranges from 5% to 40% if untreated. The human is the long-term host. **(Ref. 2,** pp. 231–237)

**177. (C)** Rocky Mountain spotted fever is the best known and most severe of tick-borne typhus diseases. Illness usually begins abruptly 2 to 12 days after tick exposure. Persistent fever is present for 2 to 3 weeks duration, with severe headache and myalgia, while nausea, vomiting, abdominal pain, and conjunctivitis occur frequently. A maculopapular rash is present in 90% of the cases, becomes petechiaie, and is accompanied by edema and cyanosis. **(Ref. 2, pp. 231–237)**

**178. (A)** Epidemic typhus is transmitted by lice. **(Ref. 2, pp. 232–239)**

**179. (B)** Regional suppurative lymphadenopathy is present in all of the diseases listed and the lesions are almost indistinguishable from each other. However, given the travel history to an endemic area, *Yersinia* should be highly suspect. **(Ref. 2, pp. 237–240)**

**180. (D)** Streptomycin is the antibiotic of choice for treatment of *Yersinia pestis*. Chloramphenicol, tetracycline, gentamycin, kanamycin, or sulfadiazine may be used as alternatives. **(Ref. 2, p. 239)**

**181. (D)** Malaria is caused by an intracellular protozoan of the species *Plasmodium.* **(Ref. 2, pp. 232–239)**

**182. (B)** Syphilis has not yet become penicillin-resistant. Treatment of tuberculosis is plagued by increasing frequency of strains with resistance to isoniazid, rifampin, and sometimes other drugs. Both enterococci and staphylococci have developed resistance to vancomycin as well as beta-lactam drugs, particularly in nosocomial infections. Some strains of enterococci have become resistant to all known antibiotics, leaving strict infection control as the only protective measure. Penicillin resistance to pneumococci has caused increased emphasis on the use of the pneumococcal vaccine. **(Ref. 61; Ref. 21)**

**183. (C)** While drug resistance has increased, there is no evidence that the infectiousness of tuberculosis organisms has increased. HIV infection greatly accelerates the progression from infection to active disease. Immigration from Asia and Latin American countries with high rates of tuberculosis has been a contributing factor (in 1994, 31.9% of reported cases with known country of origin were foreign born, of which 64.8% were in immigrants from Haiti, India, Mexico, the People's Republic of China, the Philippines, and Vietnam). Cutbacks in tuberculosis programs have been cited as another problem. Crowding and gathering of persons at risk into shared airspace occur in hospitals, nursing homes, correctional facilities and homeless shelters. (**Ref. 30**)

**184.** **(D)** In reported outbreaks, Ebola virus has caused 50% to 90% mortality. Initial clinical manifestations include fever, headache, chills, myalgia, and malaise followed by severe abdominal pain, vomiting, diarrhea, and sometimes maculopapular rash. Death is usually associated with severe hemorrhage, probably the result of disseminated intravascular coagulation (hemorrhage from multiple orifices and organ liquefaction have been anecdotally reported). Transmission occurs through contact with blood or other infected body fluids or tissues. Aerosol transmission has been demonstrated in nonhuman primates but not in humans. There is no specific treatment or vaccine. Ebola virus and the closely related Marburg virus are the only two known members of the Filovirus family. (**Ref. 30**)

**185.** **(B)** The 1993 surveillance case definition for AIDS includes all HIV-infected persons with CD4 lymphocyte counts of less than $200/mm^3$, regardless of symptoms. Persistent generalized lymphadenopathy is a common manifestation of symptomatic HIV but does not count as AIDS. Candidiasis is AIDS-defining if it is esophageal, tracheal, bronchial, or pulmonary, but not oral or vaginal. Invasive cervical carcinoma and recurrent bacterial pneumonia are AIDS-defining, but not dysplasia or recurrent bronchitis. All of the conditions listed are associated with HIV infection. AIDS does not encompass all symptomatic HIV infections or all opportunistic infections and diseases. An additional change in 1993 was the inclusion of pulmonary tuberculosis (previously, only extrapulmonary tuberculosis was AIDS-defining). (**Ref. 28**)

**186.** **(C)** Chlamydia is the STD with the highest incidence in the United States. Coinfection with gonorrhea is so prevalent that combined treatment is recommended when gonorrhea is identified. Chlamydial and gonorrheal infections are often impossible to distinguish clinically. In men, the manifestations of urethritis are indistinguishable from gonorrhea and include an opaque discharge of moderate or scanty quantity, urethral itching, and burning on urination. In women, the clinical manifestations are often extremely similar to those of gonorrhea: mucopurulent endocervical discharge with edema, erythema, and easily induced endocervical bleeding. Asymptomatic, chronic infections of the endometrium and fallopian tubes may lead to the same outcomes as symptomatic chlamydial infections: infertility or ectopic pregnancy. Unwed sexually active teenagers living in urban areas are at highest risk. (**Ref. 19,** pp. 86, 87; **Ref. 54,** pp. 104, 105)

**187.** **(E)** Mucopurulent cervicitis is a frequent clinical manifestation of chlamydial infection in the woman. Bartholinitis, perihepatitis (Fitz-Hugh-Curtis syndrome), and proctitis are less frequent manifestations but certainly well documented. Infection during pregnancy may result in conjunctival and pneumonic infection of the newborn. (**Ref. 19,** p. 87)

**188.** **(A)** It usually takes several months for untreated cryptococcal meningitis to terminate fatally. Only 8% of AIDS patients in the United States and Africa have developed cryptococcosis. Cryptococcosis is a fungal infection for which antibiotics are ineffective. Sputum cultures are positive in only 20% of cases. (**Ref. 19,** p. 110; **Ref. 2,** p. 289)

**189.** **(C)** Fatalities in the absence of dengue hemorrhagic fever are rare. Dengue is a viral disease of acute onset, spread by *Aedes aegypti* mosquitoes. There is no available active or passive immunization. (**Ref. 19,** pp. 118, 119; **Ref. 2,** p. 224)

**190.** **(D)** The Epstein-Barr virus has been associated with all of the other responses. (**Ref. 19,** pp. 291, 292)

**191.** **(B)** Although initially suspected as the cause of chronic fatigue syndrome because of boosts in EBV antibody filters, the link is now disputed. (**Ref. 19,** pp. 291, 292)

**192.** **(A)** There are three classical clinical manifestations (caused by three closely related species): cystic hydatid disease (caused by *Echinococcus granulosus*); multilocular or alveolar hydatid disease (caused by *E. multilocularis*); and polycystic hydatid disease (caused by *E. vogeli*). The lesions may be identified by CT scans, sonograms, and roentgenograms. The usual intermediate hosts are herbivores, with canines being the definitive hosts. (**Ref. 53,** pp. 148, 149)

**193.** (**A**)  All of the responses are correct except that *Dracunculus medinensis* is a large nematode, not a tapeworm. (**Ref. 19,** p. 144)

**194.** (**C**)  Light hookworm infections generally produce few or no clinical effects. (**Ref. 19,** p. 219)

**195.** (**D**)  Reservoirs for the Chinese liver fluke include humans, cats, dogs, swine, and other animals. (**Ref. 19,** p. 96)

**196.** (**C**)  The diagnostic serologic test is designed to detect *antibody* made against the surface of the virus, not antigens on the viral surface. Non-A, non-B hepatitis, the parenteral form of which recently has been attributed predominantly to hepatitis C, has been the leading cause of transfusion-associated hepatitis since at least the early 1970s. With the introduction in 1990 of voluntary blood bank screening for hepatitis C antibody (anti-HCV), relative frequency patterns may change. Unfortunately, however, a prolonged interval between exposure and onset of illness and subsequent detection of anti-HCV may limit the effectiveness of this test for screening to prevent transfusion-associated hepatitis. (**Ref. 34,** pp. 6–8)

**197.** (**E**)  Human papilloma virus (HPV) belongs to the papovavirus group of DNA viruses (the human wart viruses) unrelated to hepatitis A virus. (**Ref. 19,** p. 482)

**198.** (**C**)  Lepromatous leprosy typically produces large numbers of acid-fast organisms in the skin. The eponymal name for leprosy is Hansen's disease, not Harris' disease. The two classically described clinical manifestations of the disease are lepromatous and tuberculoid leprosy, with the etiologic agent being *Mycobacterium leprae*. The current minimal regimen recommended by the WHO for lepromatous leprosy is: rifampin, once monthly; dapsone, daily; and clofazimine, daily (with an extra large dose once a month). (**Ref. 19,** pp. 243–246)

**199.** (**A**)  Lyme disease is caused by a spirochete, not a virus. Serologic tests for *Borrelia burgdorferi,* the etiologic agent, are insensitive during the first several weeks of infection. The current first-line treatment recommendation for adults is tetracycline or doxycycline for 10 to 30 days. Antibiotic treatment in the early stages of the illness usually prevents progression to chronic disease. (**Ref. 19,** pp. 255–257; **Ref. 2,** p. 295)

**200.** (**A**) The etiologic agent of erythema infectiosum (fifth disease) is parvovirus B19, not echovirus B19. The remaining choices are correct. (**Ref. 19,** p. 159)

**201.** (**E**) CDC's recommended regimen for treatment of gonococcal infection in pregnancy is ceftriaxone (plus erythromycin instead of tetracycline for treatment of concurrent chlamydial infection). For pregnant women allergic to beta-lactams, the recommended substitution for ceftriaxone is spectinomycin. Diagnosis by culture is preferred, although a positive urethral smear with a compatible history is accepted in most clinics. (**Ref. 36,** pp. 21–24)

**202.** (**E**) The Advisory Committee on Immunization Practices guidelines clearly state that "conjugate (Hib) vaccine may be given simultaneously with diphtheria and tetanus toxoid and pertussis vaccine absorbed; combined measles, mumps, rubella vaccine; oral poliovirus vaccine; or inactivated poliovirus vaccine." Earlier recommendations to delay Hib immunization until 18 months of age are obsolete because of the availability of newer conjugated vaccines with proven effectiveness beginning at 2 months of age. (**Ref. 37,** pp. 1–7)

**203.** (**A**) The hepatitis B virus is a DNA virus. (**Ref. 38,** p. 5; **Ref. 2,** p. 133)

**204.** (**E**) All of the responses represent known complications of infection with the hepatitis B virus except gallbladder cancer. (**Ref. 38,** p. 7)

**205.** (**C**) If this patient were immune, the hepatitis B surface antibody (anti-HBs) would be positive. Anti-HBc develops in all HBV infections and persists indefinitely. It can indicate current or past HBV infection. HBsAg can be identified in serum 30 to 60 days after exposure to HBV and persists for a variable period; persistence for over 6 months is indicative of a carrier state. Anti-HBs develops after a resolved infection and is thought to be responsible for long-term immunity. The IgM core antibody develops early and persists for at least 6 months; therefore, it is helpful in identifying a recent infection. If the HBsAg is positive and IgM anti-HBc is negative, a carrier state is likely. The hepatitis B vaccine induces anti-HBs, not anti-HBc, because the antigen used in the vaccine is the surface (not core) antigen. (**Ref. 19,** pp. 200–207; **Ref. 38,** pp. 5–22)

**206.** **(E)** All of the responses are true except that most persons with HIV infection reside in developing countries including sub-Saharan Africa, Southern and Southeast Asia, Latin America, and the Caribbean. These are frightening numbers, especially the worldwide figures and particularly if one extrapolates into the 21st century. (**Ref. 39,** p. 357)

**207.** **(E)** Transfusion and blood product associated AIDS cases have stabilized at a low level. (**Ref. 39,** p. 358)

**208.** **(D)** *Pneumocystis carinii* pneumonia is the most common manifestation of AIDS, appearing in one half of AIDS patients. (**Ref. 2,** p. 118)

**209.** **(E)** In areas where travelers will be at risk of acquiring chloroquine-resistant *P. falciparum* (Asia, Africa, South America), mefloquine (a quinolone methanol) alone is recommended. According to the most current recommendations from the Centers for Disease Control, the dose (250 mg for adults) should be taken weekly, starting 1 week before travel. Prophylaxis should be continued weekly during travel in malarious areas and for 4 weeks after a person leaves such areas. (**Ref. 19,** p. 265; **Ref. 39,** p. 630)

**210.** **(D)** For grave infections or in persons needing therapy who are unable to retain oral medication, the recommended treatment is intravenous quinine. Parenteral quinidine is equally effective in treating severe malaria. (**Ref. 19,** pp. 267–268)

**211.** **(B)** Vancomycin given intravenously is the drug of choice for treatment of methicillin-resistant *S. aureus* infections. High-dose trimethoprim-sulfamethoxazole (for adults) is a useful alternative to vancomycin but is not considered the therapy of choice. A worrisome development has been the emergence of strains resistant to vancomycin as well as to methicillin. (**Ref. 20,** p. 72)

212. **(C)** Direct progression to pulmonary tuberculosis occurs in only 5% of cases following the initial infection, although it may be as high as 10% per year in HIV-infected persons. BCG vaccination is contraindicated for persons with AIDS and other symptomatic HIV infection. In the United States, extrapulmonary tuberculosis is much less common than pulmonary (although the number of cases of extrapulmonary TB has risen as a consequence of the AIDS epidemic). (**Ref. 19,** pp. 457, 462)

213. **(C)** Pulmonary tuberculosis in patients with HIV infection cannot readily be distinguished from other pulmonary infections. With some exceptions (eg, multiple-drug–resistant TB), patients with TB and HIV infection respond relatively well to standard antituberculosis drugs. Their treatment, however, should include at least four drugs initially, and the treatment may need to be longer than the usual duration. Some false-negative skin tests may be encountered in HIV-positive patients. They should be given a Mantoux skin test, however, because significant results are very meaningful. (**Ref. 40; Ref. 41**)

214. **(A)** There is no known pulmonary botulism. Food botulism is an intoxication caused by ingestion of the preformed toxin in the contaminated food. Infant botulism is caused by absorption of the toxin produced in vivo in the intestinal tract after colonization by the organism. Wound botulism results from the elaboration of the toxin in vivo after multiplication of the organism in an infected traumatized wound. The undetermined classification is used for those cases of botulism in individuals over 12 months of age in whom no food or wound source has been implicated. (**Ref. 2,** p. 197)

215. **(E)** Avocados have never been implicated in an outbreak of botulism. Vegetables are far more commonly implicated than fruits, and meats the least implicated of the three. In the United States, most cases can be traced to home-canned foods. (**Ref. 2,** p. 197)

216. **(D)** With current treatment, the fatality rate for infant botulism cases requiring hospitalization is less than 3%. (**Ref. 2,** p. 197; **Ref. 16,** pp. 1273–1276)

**217.** **(E)** SSPE is a late, rare neurologic complication of measles (not rubella). The important point to keep in mind here is that even if receiving measles vaccine is associated with SSPE in extremely rare cases, receiving measles vaccine significantly lowers risk of acquiring SSPE by protecting against measles, which before widespread immunization was a more common illness. (**Ref. 58,** pp. 234–240)

**218.** **(C)** There is no contraindication to giving the MMR and OPV vaccines (both live virus vaccines) simultaneously. (**Ref. 58,** pp. 285–287)

**219.** **(E)** WHO hopes to eradicate polio by the year 2000. As a result of the virtual eradication of wild poliovirus infection in the United States, most cases of endemic polio in this country are related to vaccination. (**Ref. 73,** p. 360)

**220.** **(A)** Pneumococcal pneumonia only accounts for 10% to 25% of all pneumonias. (**Ref. 42,** pp. 64, 65; **Ref. 19,** p. 330)

**221.** **(B)** Adults with asymptomatic or symptomatic HIV infection are listed as one of the recommended categories of adults to be vaccinated with pneumococcal vaccine. Pneumococcal vaccine is not recommended for use in children under 2 years old. (**Ref. 43,** p. 67; **Ref. 2,** p. 89)

**222.** **(C)** Legionella is frequently isolated from water sources unrelated to outbreaks of human disease. Thus routine testing of potable water systems or cooling towers is not of much value and therefore not recommended, since the organism is ubiquitous. In previous outbreaks, disease has been associated with exposure to evaporative condensers, cooling towers, showers, whirlpools, and even respiratory therapy equipment. (**Ref. 43,** p. 349)

**223.** **(C)** Figures published regularly by WHO may represent only a small percentage of the total number of cases that actually occur. In fact, many countries do not report certain communicable diseases at all. Yellow fever and occasionally cholera are the only vaccines required for travel, but others may be recommended for personal protection. (**Ref. 71,** p. 55)

**224. (A)** In general, inactivated vaccines may be administered simultaneously at different sites. Cholera, typhoid, and plague vaccines are the ones most likely to cause local or systemic side effects. Simultaneous administration of diphtheria-pertussis-tetanus (DPT), oral poliovaccine (OPV), and measles-mumps-rubella (MMR) is recommended when individuals require multiple antigens and there is doubt that the recipient will return to receive further doses of the vaccine. Unless there are time constraints, cholera and yellow fever vaccines should be administered at an interval of more than 3 weeks. If the vaccines cannot be administered at least 3 weeks apart, they should be given simultaneously. **(Ref. 71,** p. 60)

**225. (E)** If administration of Ig becomes necessary because of imminent exposure to disease, live-virus vaccine may be administered simultaneously with Ig—but with the recognition that vaccine-induced immunity may be compromised. The vaccine should be administered in a separate site from Ig inoculation. **(Ref. 71,** p. 61)

**226. (B)** Travelers must be informed that regardless of the antimalarial regimen employed, it is still possible to contract malaria. Common symptoms of malaria are headache, malaise, fever, chills, and sweats, which may occur at intervals. Neither physician nor traveler should presumptively ascribe the symptoms to a "flulike" illness. Delaying appropriate treatment can have serious or even fatal consequences. **(Ref. 72)**

**227. (A)** By undergoing mutation, the influenza virus can circumvent immunity produced by preexisting forms. **(Ref. 44,** pp. 1–15)

**228. (C)** The difficulties in controlling the snail population make it hard to eliminate schistosomiasis. **(Ref. 2,** p. 302)

**229. (A)** The major emphasis for control of this disease is to eliminate the snail. One way to do so is by improving irrigation and agricultural practices by draining and filling farm lands. **(Ref. 2,** p. 303)

**230. (A)** The common mode of transmission of the bacillus is by airborne droplet nuclei from sputum of infected individuals. **(Ref. 2,** p. 161)

**231. (D)** Diagnosis is best made by smears from a bubo. Bubonic plague is spread by the bite of infected fleas, whereas pneumonic plague can be carried by airborne droplets. Bubonic plague inflames the lymph nodes of the inguinal region and, less often, the axilla. The most effective antibiotic is streptomycin. (**Ref. 2,** p. 239)

**232. (C)** *Vibrio cholerae* proliferates within the lumen of the intestine and does not invade the bloodstream or the tissues. A powerful endotoxin is elaborated by the organism, which produces an inhibition of sodium transport by the cells of the intestinal mucosa, thus impairing its resorption capacity. The result is loss of electrolytes. The fluid loss is mainly isotonic. (**Ref. 2,** p. 176)

**233. (A)** Rhinoviruses, of which there are many recognized serotypes, plus at least one subtype, are the major known etiologic agents of the common cold in adults. (**Ref. 56**)

**234. (D)** The organisms known to be responsible for tinea pedis are members of the *Tinea* and *Epid rmophyton* genuses. (**Ref. 4,** pp. 318–321)

**235. (B)** Ascariasis is transmitted by vehicles such as water, food, milk, serum, or plasma. (**Ref. 19,** pp. 50–52)

**236. (C)** If body temperature is affected by staphylococcal food poison, it will probably be subnormal. (**Ref. 56**)

**237. (E)** When the subject is epidemics and pandemics, influenza is at the forefront. It is known to cause mortality among predicted high-risk groups (infants, young children, and those over 65). An epidemic causes excessive morbidity but low mortality. Because of the periodic-cyclic recurrence, epidemiologists can forecast (with limited accuracy) future epidemic patterns and predict the likely prevalent virus type. Winter prevalence is most likely. (**Ref. 45,** pp. 1–15)

**238. (E)** Other diseases that might require complete or modified quarantine are cholera, meningococcal meningitis, and epidemic typhus. (**Ref. 19**)

**239. (A)** This form of malaria is a sudden, severe disease. The developmental cycle is the same as vivax malaria—48 hours—but the chills and fever come at irregular intervals. The cerebral symptoms, biliary remittent fever, and shock are caused by the parasites plugging capillaries. Hemoglobinuria is caused by extensive hemolysis. (**Ref. 2,** p. 240)

**240.** (**E**)  The occurrence of meningococcal meningitis is worldwide. The disease is most prevalent in the winter and spring. The male child and young adult are more likely to have the infection than their female counterparts. However, it could be more common in adults if they live under crowded conditions, such as in barracks and institutions. The reservoir is human. (**Ref. 19,** pp. 280–284)

**241.** (**D**)  The case fatality rate for leptospirosis is generally low but increases with advancing age and may reach up to 20% in patients with jaundice and kidney damage who have not been treated with renal dialysis; deaths are due predominantly to hepatorenal failure, adult respiratory distress syndrome, or cardiac arrhythmias secondary to myocardial involvement. Although pathogenic leptospiroses are considered to be members of one species, *Leptospira interrogans,* about 20 serogroups, including more than 170 serovars, have been identified antigenically. Leptospirosis is sometimes considered to be a group of diseases. (**Ref. 19,** p. 247)

**242.** (**E**)  Person-to-person transmission of the disease is rare. (**Ref. 19,** p. 248)

**243.** (**D**)  Leukopenia, not leukocytosis, appears early and is most pronounced during the first week of illness. (**Ref. 19,** pp. 486–488)

**244.** (**C**)  The first sign of trichinosis is a sudden appearance of edema of the upper eyelids. Shortly thereafter, muscle soreness and pain, skin lesions, thirst, profuse sweating, chills, weakness, prostration, and eosinophilia appear. Respiratory and neurologic symptoms may develop 3 to 6 weeks after onset. (**Ref. 19,** pp. 446)

**245.** (**C**)  Skeletal muscle biopsy, approximately 10 days after exposure, would give conclusive evidence of infection; however, skin test, eosinophilia, flocculation, and complement fixation tests may help in diagnosis. (**Ref. 19,** p. 446)

**246.** **(E)** The main source of transmission is eating food that contains raw or insufficiently cooked pork; therefore, prevention would be to properly cook pork. Heating to a temperature of 65.5°C (150°F) or cooling to –25°C (–13°F) for 10 days will destroy the cysts, which are not visible to a meat inspector. **(Ref. 19, pp. 447, 448)**

**247.** **(E)** Cholera is an acute specific infection of the alimentary tract caused by the cholera vibrio. The major characteristics are sudden onset; profuse, watery stools; watery vomiting; rapid dehydration; muscular cramps; suppression of urine; and collapse. **(Ref. 2, p. 178)**

**248.** **(D)** The mode of transmission is by fecal-oral spread, infected water, and food. Milk is not a common component of the diet in the countries where cholera prevails. **(Ref. 2, p. 260)**

**249.** **(B)** Tularemia is a fatal bacteremia of rabbits and certain rodents and secondarily an accidental infection of domestic animals and humans. The common characteristics are a sudden and dramatic onset of chills, fever, headache, and vomiting. The primary lesion usually ulcerates. **(Ref. 2, p. 260)**

**250.** **(B)** All of the responses are correct except person-to-person transmission. Tularemia has also been acquired by eating poorly cooked wild rabbits or hares or by bites of infected animals and occasionally by inhaling contaminated dust. **(Ref. 2, p. 260)**

**251.** **(C)** Sometimes confused with measles (rubeola), scarlet fever, or both, rubella (German measles) is a mild febrile infectious disease with a maculopapular rash. **(Ref. 2, p. 70)**

**252.** **(D)** The most dangerous period for a pregnant woman is during the first 3 months of pregnancy. Therefore, if a woman who has not had rubella wishes to become pregnant, she should wait 2 months after being vaccinated to do so. **(Ref. 2, p. 71)**

**253.** **(B)** While it is possible to vomit or have diarrhea coincidentally with the other symptoms, gastrointestinal disturbances are not part of the usual illness complex. **(Ref. 2, p. 71)**

**254.** **(B)** Milk and milk products are principle vehicles for typhoid fever. **(Ref. 19, pp.** 469–474)

**255.** **(D)** When a group of individuals comes down with typhoid fever, you must determine what caused the outbreak. This can only be done by interviewing those who participated in the event that led to the outbreak. **(Ref. 19, pp.** 469–474)

**256.** **(A)** Measles (rubeola) is a common childhood disease, occurring in 90% or more of the nonimmunized population. **(Ref. 2, p.** 65)

**257.** **(B)** In the United States, death from measles (rubeola) is rare. The greater concern is for the secondary bacterial infections that occur. **(Ref. 2, p.** 65)

**258.** **(C)** Only *Mycobacterium tuberculosis* and *M. bovis* are causative agents of human tuberculosis. The others are causes of "atypical" mycobacterial infections. **(Ref. 2, p.** 159)

**259.** **(C)** The disease is easily transmitted by dusty fomites, and then spores are inhaled. **(Ref. 19, pp.** 98–100)

**260.** **(A)** This mycotic infection is extremely common in scattered highly endemic arid and semiarid areas of the Western Hemisphere and is sometimes called valley fever after the Central Valley of California, an endemic area. Common symptoms are fever, chills, cough, and pleural pain. **(Ref. 19, pp.** 98–100)

**261.** **(E)** Infection can occur in humans, cattle, cats, dogs, horses, burros, sheep, swine, wild desert rodents, coyotes, chinchillas, llamas, and other species. Insects are not reservoirs or vectors. **(Ref. 19, pp.** 98–100)

**262.** **(D)** Darkfield microscopic examination can detect primary and secondary syphilis but is useless in late-lesion syphilis. The major means for diagnosis of syphilis is by various forms of serologic tests. **(Ref. 2, p.** 111)

**263.** **(C)** In the United States it is recommended that the diphtheria-pertussis-tetanus (DPT) vaccine be given at 2, 4, 6, and 15 to 18 months with a booster at school entry, but not after the seventh birthday. The pertussis portion of DPT is contraindicated in older children and adults. **(Ref. 19, pp.** 319, 320)

**264. (A)** The transmission of meningococcal meningitis is maintained by person-to-person transfer. There is no extrahuman reservoir. The meningococcus dies quickly outside the body when exposed to drying or sunlight. Overcrowded living conditions allow for nasopharyngeal secretions to be passed from one individual to another. (**Ref. 19,** pp. 280–284)

**265. (C)** Malaria resistance to most anti-malarial drugs has become very high in Thailand. Doxycycline is recommended for prophylactic use at this time. (**Ref. 2,** pp. 246–247)

**266. (D)** Proguanil by itself has too high a resistance to be considered a good treatment option in a patient with this history. Clinical malaria developing in the face of chemosuppression suggests probable drug resistance for which the cinchona alkaloids (quinine and quinidine) and pyrimethamine-sulfadoxine (Fansidar) are probably the best options. Chloroquine in sufficient doses may also be useful. (**Ref. 2,** pp. 246–249)

**267. (D)** All of these are sexually transmitted diseases. (**Ref. 56,** p. 411)

**268. (D)** Early syphilis is considered transmittable, whereas late syphilis is rarely infectious. In contrast with the lesions of early syphilis, considerable destruction accompanies late lesions. Primary syphilis is usually detected by darkfield microscopy, whereas late syphilis is by serologic test and spinal fluid examination. Penicillin treatment is indicated in both, but neurosyphilis requires more extensive treatment regimens, and tissue damage from tertiary syphilis may be irreversible. (**Ref. 56,** pp. 528–532)

**269. (D)** Passive immunization denotes the provision of temporary immunity and the administration of preformed antitoxin or antibodies. Maternal antibodies are an example of passive immunization. Active immunization denotes the production of antibodies or antitoxin in response to the administration of a vaccine or a toxoid. (**Ref. 45**)

**270. (D)** Adjuvants are usually aluminum compounds, which are used to enhance the immunogenicity of the vaccine. Vaccines containing antigens must be injected deeply into muscle mass, since subcutaneous administration may cause local irritation and even necrosis. Mercurials and specific antibiotics are used to inhibit or even prevent bacterial growth in viral culture or in the final product. (Ref. 45, p. 208)

271. (C) Killed vaccines have not been associated with fetal risk. There is no risk to the fetus from passive immunization of pregnant women with immune globulin, and experience has not revealed any risk to the fetus when the mother is immunized with polio vaccine. (Ref. 45, pp. 222, 223)

272. (E) Permethrin 5% cream is now widely considered to be the therapy of choice for scabies. It is at least as effective as 1% lindane and more effective than crotamiton and topical sulfur ointment. It is recommended before lindane, since it appears to be a significantly safer treatment. A 1% permethrin shampoo is recommended for head lice but not for scabies. Lindane 1% lotion and cream have been widely used for scabies, but the shampoo is likewise intended for pediculosis, not for scabies. (Ref. 65, p. 21)

273. (D) Toxoplasmosis is a systemic protozoan disease. A primary infection during the early gestational period of pregnancy may lead to death of the fetus or to chorioretinitis, brain damage with cerebral calcification, and macrocephaly or hydrocephaly. (Ref. 21, p. 431)

274. (E) Histoplasmosis is a systemic mycosis of varying severity, with the primary lesion usually in the lungs. The infectious agent is *Histoplasma capsulatum,* a dimorphic fungus, growing as a mold in soil and as a yeast in animals and the human host. A common mode of transmission is by inhalation of airborne spores in dust. (Ref. 56, pp. 323, 344)

275. (A) Genital herpes is a viral disease that may be chronic and recurring and for which no known cure exists. Systemic acyclovir treatment provides partial control of the symptoms and signs of herpes episodes; it accelerates healing but does not eradicate the infection or affect the subsequent risk, frequency, or severity of recurrences after the drug is discontinued. Topical therapy with acyclovir is substantially less effective than therapy with the oral drug. (Ref. 36, p. 16)

**276.** **(A)** Nosocomial infections, despite our current control methods, still occur at a proportion of 5 to 10 per hundred of all US hospital admissions. **(Ref. 2,** pp. 203–205)

**277.** **(D)** An incubation period this short (5 minutes to 2 hours) almost certainly represents chemical food poisoning, since even staphylococcal food intoxication (preformed toxin), with its abrupt and sometimes violent onset, ordinarily has an incubation period of 30 minutes to 7 hours, usually 2 to 4 hours. In this case, the incriminated chemical was zinc, which is a major constituent of galvanized metal. On contact with acidic foods and beverages, it is converted to zinc salts, which are readily absorbed by the body. **(Ref. 46)**

**278.** **(D)** Influenza vaccine is only recommended for the following categories of children: those with chronic disorders of the pulmonary or cardiovascular systems, including children with asthma; those who have required regular medical follow-up or hospitalization during the preceding year because of chronic metabolic diseases (including diabetes mellitus), renal dysfunction, hemoglobinopathies, or immunosuppression (including medication-induced immunosuppression); and children and teenagers (6 months to 18 years of age) who are receiving long-term aspirin therapy and therefore may be at risk of developing Reye's syndrome after influenza. **(Ref. 45,** p. 3; **Ref. 46)**

**279.** **(B)** Pneumococcal vaccine is not recommended for routine use in healthy children. It is recommended for certain groups of children at high risk of pneumococcal disease, including those with decreased immune function and certain chronic diseases. **(Ref. 43)**

**280.** **(C)** HIV transmission from routine daily household contact with an HIV-infected person is extremely rare, unless there is blood exposure. **(Ref. 19,** p. 3)

**281.** **(C)** Stool smears in giardiasis usually show only few or no leukocytes. Transmission is by ingestion of cysts, which may be water- or food-borne. Usual concentrations of chlorine in water treatment do not kill giardia cysts. Filtration can be effective. Stools are usually greasy and foul-smelling. **(Ref. 2,** pp. 186, 187)

**282. (D)** In the United States, most hepatitis B transmission is probably sexual. Acute transfusion-associated cases are now rare. About 10% to 15% of persons reported with HBV infection have been identified as parenteral drug abusers. Delta hepatitis can only infect persons also infected with hepatitis B and particularly affects drug users. Control of hepatitis B among intravenous drug abusers and persons in other high-risk groups is critical for limiting the spread of HBV and delta virus in the general population. Many HBV outbreaks have been demonstrated among intravenous drug abusers over the past two decades, and serologic surveys have demonstrated that HBV infection is highly prevalent in this group. **(Ref. 47)**

**283. (D)** It is estimated that in approximately 20% to 40% of cases of maternal HIV infection, the virus is transmitted vertically to the infant. Administering zidovudine (AZT) prenatally to the infected mother and postnatally to the infant has been reported to reduce this substantially. **(Ref. 2, p. 118)**

**284. (C)** Chancroid is fairly common but one of the least important of the sexually transmitted diseases. **(Ref. 19, pp. 81–83)**

**285. (B)** Although sexual contact is the most common mode of transmission, other modes, such as contaminated clothing, douching equipment, or enema nozzles have been known to transmit the disease. **(Ref. 19, pp. 259–261)**

**286. (D)** Gonorrhea can be difficult to diagnose, especially in women and in chronic cases; furthermore, only a small fraction of cases are reported. The human is the only known reservoir. **(Ref. 19, pp. 185–190)**

**287. (E)** Bacterial vaginosis is one of the common types of vaginitis. Physicians should familiarize themselves with this syndrome, because it causes women a great deal of discomfort. Treatment is metronidazole, 500 mg by mouth twice a day for 7 days. Formerly attributed to *Gardnerella* organisms, anaerobes are now considered to be involved in pathogenesis. Partners are not routinely treated. **(Ref. 36)**

**288. (D)** Trichomoniasis. Male sexual partners of women with trichomoniasis should be treated similarly. Metronidazole is contraindicated in the first trimester of pregnancy and is preferably avoided throughout pregnancy. (**Ref. 36**)

**289.** (**C**) Podophyllin is the treatment of choice for condyloma acuminata. (**Ref. 36,** pp. 18–20)

**290.** (**A**) Chancroid may be a more common cause of genital ulcers than is currently recognized. A first-line drug regimen is erythromycin, 500 mg orally four times a day for 7 days. (**Ref. 36**)

**291.** (**B**) Doxycycline 100 mg PO b.i.d. for 21 days is the treatment of choice for lymphogranuloma venereum. (**Ref. 36,** p. 15)

**292.** (**B**) Tetanus (lockjaw) is an acute disease brought about by toxin of the tetanus bacillus growing anaerobically at the site of injury. Common characteristics are painful muscular contractions, mainly in the masseter and neck muscles and secondarily in the trunk muscles. Fatality rates vary from 30% to 90% (in the absence of effective immunization). The best protection is by active immunization with tetanus toxoid. (**Ref. 19,** pp. 430–435)

**293.** (**A**) Rabies usually develops into fatal acute encephalomyelitis. It progresses to paresis or paralysis. The incubation period is usually 2 to 8 weeks, depending on the extent of the laceration and location. (**Ref. 19,** pp. 353–362)

**294.** (**D**) Leptospirosis is a group of zoonotic spirochetal diseases with protean manifestations. The usual characteristics are fever, headache, chills, severe malaise, vomiting, muscular aches, and conjunctivitis, and infrequently, renal insufficiency and jaundice. Fatality rates increase with age and reach 20% or more in patients with renal involvement and jaundice. (**Ref. 19,** pp. 247–250)

**295.** (**E**) Mice are a common carrier for this virus. The characteristics are diversified, with influenzalike attacks or meningeal symptoms. The virus is transmitted by excreted urine, saliva, and feces, in food or dust eaten by humans. (**Ref. 19,** pp. 257–259)

**296.** (**C**); **297.** (**A**); **298.** (**A**); **299.** (**D**); **300.** (**B**) Short incubation periods are characteristic of outbreaks of chemical etiology (incubation in minutes rather than hours) and staphylococcal intoxication (incubation period mostly less than 6 hours). Infectious hepatitis A has an incubation period of up to several weeks. Outbreaks of *Clostridium perfringens* are recognized readily but confirmed with difficulty because of problems involved in the transport of aerobic specimens during culture. Outbreaks of mushroom poisoning from amanita toxin are likely to be reported because of their seriousness, but because of their rarity, they may not be recognized. *Vibrio parahaemolyticus* from ingesting raw fish is less often considered clinically, epidemiologically, and in the laboratory, and is not so likely to be confirmed. (**Ref. 69**)

301. (D); 302. (E); 303. (B); 304. (A); 305. (C)  Outbreaks of botulism are frequently involved with home preserved vegetables and, in Alaska, fish. *C. perfringens* outbreaks usually involve beef, as do staphylococcal outbreaks. Salmonella outbreaks are caused by many different vehicles, including meat, poultry, dairy products, and salads. Ciguatera outbreaks involve mainly coral reef fish, particularly grouper; and *T. spiralis* outbreaks usually involve pork and sausage. Paralytic shellfish poisonings are frequently associated with the consumption of clams. (**Ref. 69**)

306. (A)  Anthrax has a worldwide distribution affecting cloven-hoofed animals. Cases of human disease are sporadic and can be traced to the handling of infected animals or animal products. (**Ref. 19,** pp. 17–20)

307. (D)  Brucellosis has a worldwide distribution. The reservoir for the *Brucella* organism is directly related to the specific animal husbandry practiced; bovine (*B. abortus*), porcine (*B. suis*), and caprine (*B. militensus*). (**Ref. 19,** pp. 66–68)

308. (C)  Eradication of the carrier state is often difficult and may involve multiple courses of various antibiotics. (**Ref. 19,** pp. 414, 415)

309. (E)  The definition includes any hospital-acquired infections, including ones acquired from employees or environmental sources. (**Ref. 19,** p. 504)

310. (B)  All responses are important in infection control, but hand washing is the single most important procedure for preventing nosocomial infections. (**Ref. 60**)

**311.** **(C)** A full series of the hepatitis B vaccine should be given to all infants born to HBsAg-positive mothers, and the first dose should be given concurrently with HBIg (but at a different site). Subsequent doses of hepatitis B vaccine should be given as recommended for the specific vaccine. (**Ref. 38,** p. 18)

**312.** **(C)** Paralytic shellfish poisoning (PSP) is caused by ingestion of bivalve mollusks (most often oysters, clams, mussels) that feed on toxin-producing dinoflagellates. Characteristic symptoms are paresthesias of mouth, lips, face, and extremities. In severe cases dysphagia, muscle weakness, or frank paralysis, ataxia, and respiratory insufficiency may occur. Treatment is supportive, but PSP may be fatal even in previously healthy people. The incubation period is 5 minutes to 4 hours. PSP occurs seasonally in summer and fall, often in association with a red tide. Prevention is to ensure shellfish come from safe waters. Toxin-contaminated food tastes and appears normal. The toxin (saxitoxin) is heat stable so cooking provides no protection. (**Ref. 64,** pp. 893–901)

**313.** **(D)** Specific treatment involves intravenous and intrathecal administration of amphotericin B and miconazole in conjunction with oral rifampin. Recoveries have been rare despite the organism's being sensitive to antibiotics in laboratory studies. No specific vaccine is available. (**Ref. 16,** pp. 286–288)

**314.** **(D)** In the United States rabies has decreased in both humans and domestic animals. In 1950, 4979 cases of rabies were reported among dogs and 18 in humans. In 1989, 160 cases were reported among dogs and 1 in humans. The disease in wildlife, especially skunks, foxes, raccoons, and bats, has become more prevalent. Only Hawaii remains consistently rabies free. Treatment of choice is human diploid cell rabies vaccine (HDCV); this and human rabies immune globulin (HRIG) constitute the two types of immunizing products. Both types should be used concurrently for rabies postexposure prophylaxis. Preexposure prophylaxis is available using three doses of HDCV given days 0, 7, 21, or 28. (**Ref. 42**)

**315.** **(C)** The incubation period for *Salmonella* infections is from 6 to 72 hours, usually about 12 to 36 hours. (**Ref. 19,** p. 383)

**316.** **(C)** Foods that most commonly transmit *Salmonella* infections are commercially processed meat products, inadequately cooked poultry or poultry products, raw sausages, uncooked or lightly cooked foods containing eggs or egg products, unpasteurized milk or dairy products including dried milk, and foods contaminated by an infected food handler. (**Ref. 16,** p. 382)

**317.** **(B)** Fruits and vegetables are not often identified as vehicles for *Salmonella* infection; however, in 1990 and 1991 several outbreaks of *Salmonella* were associated with cantaloupes and tomatoes. It is true that a single *Salmonella* contaminated egg can cause outbreaks of severe illness and that a *Salmonella* infection can be fatal in an otherwise healthy person if a sufficient dose is ingested. Thorough cooking kills *Salmonella,* although when eggs are heavily contaminated, standard cooking methods for many egg-containing foods may not kill all *Salmonella.* When egg-associated *Salmonella* infections occur, investigation of outbreaks and notification of state and federal agricultural departments is crucial to identify sources of contaminated eggs and to develop and implement control measures. (**Ref. 56; Ref. 52**)

**318.** **(E)** In adults it usually takes 2 weeks for antibodies to develop after receiving the influenza vaccine. In high-risk individuals vaccinated during an outbreak of influenza A, it is appropriate to use amantadine during those 2 weeks as prophylaxis. Amantadine hydrochloride is highly effective in preventing influenza caused by type A viruses, but it is not effective against type B viruses. Chemoprophylaxis is not a substitute for vaccination. Amantadine is more likely to cause troublesome side effects in older persons but seldom causes them in healthy young adults. When the normal adult dose of 200 mg is reduced to 100 mg in individuals 65 years or older, the incidence and severity of side effects decreases substantially. To be fully effective amantadine must be taken daily for the duration of influenza activity in the community. (**Ref. 45**)

**319.** **(D)** Bubonic plague is commonly transmitted by the bite of an infected flea. Other less common modes of transmission are by handling infected tissues or from contact with purulence from infected animals. The infectious agent is *Yersinia pestis*. Plague continues to be a threat in areas with persistent wild rodent infection, such as in the western third of the United States. This disease is characterized in humans chiefly by lymphadenitis and septicemia. Lymph nodes are swollen, inflamed, tender, and may suppurate. The incubation period is from 2 to 6 days. (**Ref. 19,** pp. 324–329)

**320.** (B)   If therapy is begun within 8 to 24 hours after onset, streptomycin, tetracyclines, and chloramphenicol are highly effective. Active immunization with a killed bacterial vaccine is available. Chemoprophylaxis is recommended for close contacts of confirmed or suspected plague pneumonia cases. (**Ref. 19,** p. 328)

**321.** (D)   Humans are the only reservoir for pertussis (whooping cough). Transmission is by direct contact with respiratory secretions by the airborne route, probably by droplets. It is most contagious during the early catarrhal stage and has an incubation period of 7 to 10 days. (**Ref. 19,** p. 320)

**322.** (B)   When diphtheria is suspected, one should administer antitoxin immediately after bacteriologic specimens are taken, without waiting for bacteriologic confirmation. Both penicillin and erythromycin are effective against the organism, but not as a substitute for antitoxin. If carrier states are identified they should be treated. (**Ref. 19,** p. 141)

**323.** (D)   Brucellosis (undulant fever) is usually passed to humans by diseased domestic animals such as cattle, swine, sheep, goats, horses, reindeer, and sometimes dogs. Human infections come from contact with infected tissue, blood, urine, vaginal discharges, aborted fetuses, and placentas, and by ingestion of infected milk or dairy products such as cheese. Dengue fever is transmitted by the bite of infected mosquitoes, coccidioidomycosis by inhalation of dust, onchocerciasis by the bite of infected female black flies, leishmaniasis through the bite of infected sand flies. (**Ref. 19,** pp. 67, 99, 119, 242, 309)

**324.** (E)   Positive tuberculin reactions in BCG-vaccinated persons usually indicate infection with *Mycobacterium tuberculosis*. The TB skin test should be interpreted using the standard guidelines and the patient evaluated for preventive therapy. The Mantoux method of administering the TB test is preferred over the multiple puncture devices. The absence of a reaction to the TB test does not exclude the diagnosis of TB. A number of conditions may decrease or eliminate the reaction. In persons exposed to active TB, persons with a chest roentgenogram suggestive of old inactive TB, and persons with HIV infection, a 5-mm reaction should be considered significant. (**Ref. 55,** pp. 11–15)

**325. (B)**

| Abbreviation | Term | Comments |
|---|---|---|
| HBV | Hepatitis B virus | Surface antigen of HBV |
| HBsAg | HB surface antigen | Surface antigen of HBV detectable in large quantity of serum; correlates with HBV |
| Anti-HBs | Antibody to HBsAg | Indicates past infection with and immunity to HBV, passive antibody from HBIg vaccine, or immune response from HBV vaccine |
| IgM anti-HBc | IgM class antibody to HBcAg | Indicates recent infection with HBV; positive for 4–6 months after infection |

(**Ref. 75,** p. 317)

# 3

# Noncommunicable and Chronic Diseases

**DIRECTIONS:** Each of the numbered items or incomplete statements in this section is followed by answers or completions of the statement. Select the **ONE** lettered answer or completion that is **BEST** in each case.

326. Which of the following diseases is **LEAST** likely to be preventable with lifestyle change?
    A. Cardiovascular disease
    B. Cancer
    C. Tuberculosis
    D. Chronic obstructive pulmonary disease
    E. Cirrhosis

327. Which of the following has the lowest all-age mortality rate?
    A. Single man
    B. Divorced man
    C. Widowed woman
    D. Married woman
    E. Widowed man

328. All of the following are associated with a higher risk of disease **EXCEPT**
    A. having a low socioeconomic status
    B. being female

C. having few friends
D. moving from one place to another frequently
E. being divorced

329. Of the following risk factors, which contributes the most to overall mortality?
   A. Depression and injury
   B. Overnutrition and substance abuse
   C. Alcohol and tobacco
   D. Handguns and violence
   E. Elevated cholesterol and obesity

330. Which of the following risk factors is associated with the greatest number of cancer deaths?
   A. Diet
   B. Alcohol
   C. Smoking
   D. Obesity
   E. Environmental exposures

331. Of the many risk factors for cardiovascular diseases, which three risk factors contribute the most to premature death?
   A. Smoking, diet, obesity
   B. High blood pressure, smoking, serum cholesterol
   C. Serum cholesterol, smoking, inactivity
   D. High blood pressure, smoking, stress
   E. Inactivity, stress, obesity

332. Which of the following is true for smokers in comparison with nonsmokers?
   A. A twofold increased risk of a myocardial infarction
   B. A twofold increased risk of chronic obstructive pulmonary disease
   C. A twofold increased risk of lung cancer
   D. A twofold increased risk of bladder cancer
   E. A twofold increased risk of kidney cancer

**333.** What is the most significant risk factor predisposing an individual to peripheral vascular occlusive disease?
  **A.** Diet
  **B.** Cigarette smoking
  **C.** Lack of exercise
  **D.** Age
  **E.** Diabetes mellitus

**334.** What percentage of all coronary heart disease (CHD) deaths are attributable to smoking?
  **A.** 0% to 10%
  **B.** 10% to 20%
  **C.** 20% to 30%
  **D.** 30% to 40%
  **E.** 40 to 50%

**335.** The Centers for Disease Control and Prevention have defined the fetal tobacco syndrome as including all of the following **EXCEPT**
  **A.** the mother smoked five or more cigarettes a day throughout the pregnancy
  **B.** the mother had no evidence of hypertension during pregnancy, specifically, no preeclampsia, with documentation of normal blood pressure at least once after the first trimester
  **C.** the newborn infant had symmetrical growth retardation at term, defined as birth weight less than 2500 g and a ponderal index (weight in grams divided by length) greater than 2.32
  **D.** there is no obvious cause of intrauterine growth retardation, such as congenital malformation or infection
  **E.** placental to birth weight ratio is smaller than average

**336.** All of the following are associated with the excess mortality of chronic heavy drinkers **EXCEPT**
  **A.** suicide
  **B.** cancer of the larynx
  **C.** accidents
  **D.** pneumonia
  **E.** tuberculosis

**337.** The median value for annual alcohol consumption in all 50 states of the United States is?
  **A.** 1 liter
  **B.** 3 liters

C. 7 liters
D. 10 liters
E. 15 liters

338. Among the eight geographic areas of the world, the highest median levels per capita consumption of alcohol are in which three?
    A. Africa, South America, and Europe
    B. South America, Europe, North America
    C. Asia, Africa, Central America
    D. North America, Central America, South America
    E. Australia and New Zealand, North America, Europe

339. Which of the following is **NOT** included in the 1988 Alcoholic Beverage Labeling Act?
    A. Women should not drink alcoholic beverages during pregnancy because of the risk of birth defects
    B. Consumption of alcoholic beverages may cause cancer
    C. Consumption of alcoholic beverages impairs the ability to drive a car
    D. Consumption of alcoholic beverages impairs the ability to operate machinery
    E. Consumption of alcoholic beverages may cause health problems

340. Which segment of our population has **NOT** experienced improved health over the past 30 years?
    A. Geriatric population
    B. Adult population
    C. Adolescents
    D. Children
    E. Newborn children

341. Which of the following classes of drugs of abuse typically does **NOT** cause a withdrawal syndrome?
    A. Narcotics
    B. Depressants
    C. Hallucinogens
    D. Stimulants
    E. Cannabis

**342.** Which of the following risk factors is **NOT** associated with initiation of drug abuse in adolescents or young adults?
  **A.** Parents' drug use
  **B.** Family strife
  **C.** Poor school grades
  **D.** Marriage
  **E.** Low socioeconomic status

**343.** Adoption studies have established that all of the following are at increased risk for alcoholism **EXCEPT**
  **A.** daughters of alcoholic fathers
  **B.** daughters of alcoholic mothers
  **C.** sons of alcoholic fathers
  **D.** sons of alcoholic mothers
  **E.** siblings of alcoholic children

**344.** All of the following criteria are helpful in selecting and applying a screening test **EXCEPT**
  **A.** the disease should be relatively common
  **B.** the mortality or morbidity of the untreated condition should be substantial
  **C.** an effective therapy for the presymptomatic stage is not necessary
  **D.** the screening test must be suitable for routine application
  **E.** the test should ideally have high specificity and sensitivity

**Questions 345–348:**
Use the following information regarding breast cancer to answer.

| | Breast Cancer Present | Breast Cancer Absent | Total |
|---|---|---|---|
| # women with positive mammograms | 15 | 22 | 37 |
| # women with negative mammograms | 13 | 25 | 38 |
| **Total** | 28 | 47 | 75 |

**345.** The sensitivity of the above data is expressed as

A. $\dfrac{25}{25+22} \times 100$

B. $\dfrac{15}{15+25} \times 100$

C. $\dfrac{25}{25+15} \times 100$

D. $\dfrac{15}{15+13} \times 100$

E. $\dfrac{15}{25+13} \times 100$

**346.** The specificity of the above data is expressed as

A. $\dfrac{25}{25+22} \times 100$

B. $\dfrac{25}{25+15} \times 100$

C. $\dfrac{15}{15+25} \times 100$

D. $\dfrac{15}{15+13} \times 100$

E. $\dfrac{15}{25+22} \times 100$

**347.** The positive predictive value is expressed as

A. $\dfrac{15}{15+13} \times 100$

B. $\dfrac{15}{15+22} \times 100$

C. $\dfrac{25}{25+13} \times 100$

D. $\dfrac{25}{25+22} \times 100$

E. $\dfrac{25}{15+13} \times 100$

**348.** The negative predictive value is expressed as

A. $\dfrac{15}{15+13} \times 100$

B. $\dfrac{15}{15+22} \times 100$

C. $\dfrac{25}{25+13} \times 100$

D. $\dfrac{25}{25+22} \times 100$

E. $\dfrac{25}{15+13} \times 100$

**Questions 349 and 350:**
Use the following graph to answer.

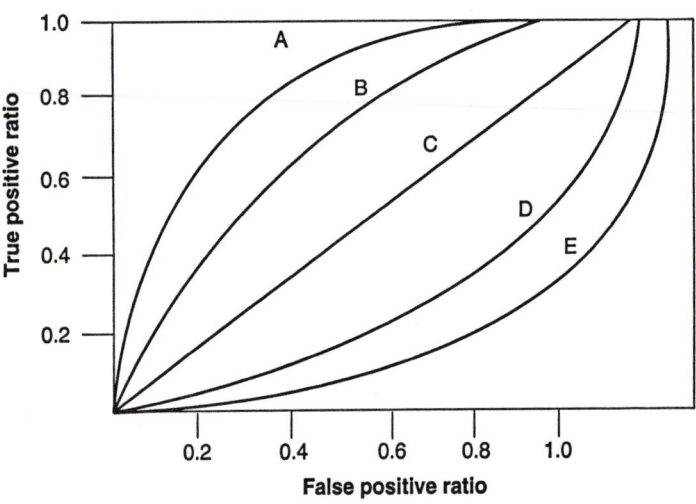

**349.** Which of the curves demonstrates the highest degree of sensitivity for each point along the abscissa?

A. Curve A
B. Curve B
C. Curve C
D. Curve D
E. Curve E

**350.** Which of the curves demonstrates the highest degree of specificity for each point along the ordinate?
 **A.** Curve A
 **B.** Curve B
 **C.** Curve C
 **D.** Curve D
 **E.** Curve E

**351.** List in order of decreasing frequency the five most common cancers in men in the United States.
 **A.** Lung, colon, prostate, bladder, rectum
 **B.** Lung, bladder, prostate, colon, rectum
 **C.** Prostate, lung, colon, bladder, rectum
 **D.** Prostate, lung, colon, rectum, bladder
 **E.** Prostate, lung, bladder, colon, rectum

**352.** List in order of decreasing frequency the five most common cancers in women in the United States.
 **A.** Breast, lung, colon, uterus, ovary
 **B.** Lung, breast, colon, uterus, ovary
 **C.** Lung, breast, ovary, colon, uterus
 **D.** Breast, lung, ovary, colon, uterus
 **E.** Lung, ovary, breast, colon, uterus

**Questions 353–359:**
Match the following risk factors with the most closely associated disease.

 **A.** diets rich in animal products
 **B.** nitrosamine preserved foods
 **C.** hepatitis B virus
 **D.** chemical irritants
 **E.** Epstein-Barr virus
 **F.** cytomegalovirus
 **G.** human papilloma virus

**353.** Colon cancer

**354.** Rectal cancer

**355.** Lung and laryngeal cancer

**356.** Stomach cancer

**357.** Nasopharyngeal cancer

**358.** Liver cancer

**359.** Cervical cancer

**Questions 360 and 361:**
A 72-year-old man has a 1-month history of angina occurring at rest, lasting up to 20 minutes. He states that the episodes have been increasing in frequency and intensity over the last several weeks. He has smoked 2 packs of cigarettes per day for 50 years and has been treated for hypertension for the last 15 years.

**360.** Which type of angina best describes this patient's pain?
  **A.** Chronic stable angina pectoris
  **B.** Variant or Prinzmetal's angina
  **C.** Silent ischemia
  **D.** Unstable angina pectoris
  **E.** Traditional angina

**361.** The initial step in management of this patient should be
  **A.** admission to the hospital for further work-up
  **B.** observation for several hours in the emergency room until pain resolves
  **C.** obtain ECG and follow patient on outpatient basis if ECG is normal
  **D.** place patient on aspirin 325 mg per day, and instruct patient to follow up in your office in 2 days
  **E.** reassure patient and send home without follow-up

**Questions 362–364:**
A 14-year-old black youth presents to your office with fever and painful joints for the past week. He also complains of a nonproductive cough and sore throat for the past week.

**362.** Appropriate initial steps for this patient should include
  **A.** throat culture for group A streptococcus
  **B.** throat culture for *Haemophilus influenza*
  **C.** roentgenograms of involved joints

    **D.** attempt at aspiration of joints
    **E.** ESR

**363.** The treatment of choice is
    **A.** doxycycline
    **B.** clindamycin
    **C.** rocephin
    **D.** penicillin
    **E.** augmentin

**364.** Possible complications include
    **A.** anemia, thrombocytopenia
    **B.** dermatomyositis, polymyositis
    **C.** hematuria, proteinuria, RBC casts
    **D.** macrocytosis or target cell formation
    **E.** polyuria, polydipsia

**Questions 365 and 366:**

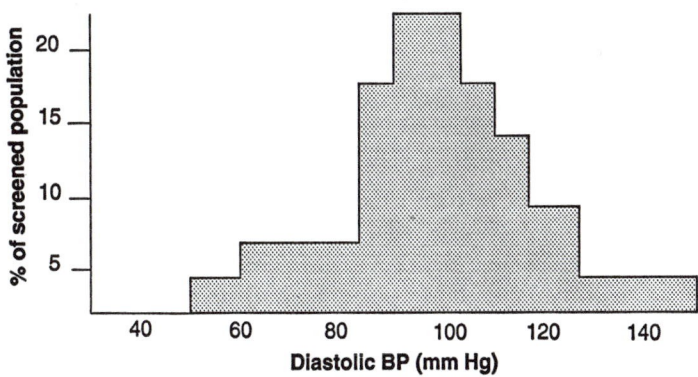

**365.** According to the above distribution for diastolic blood pressure, what is the modal value in mm Hg?
    **A.** 60 to 70
    **B.** 70 to 80
    **C.** 80 to 90
    **D.** 90 to 100
    **E.** 100 to 110

**366.** According to the above distribution, which of the following is correct?

   **A.** A majority of the screened individuals exhibit at least mild to moderate hypertension

   **B.** A majority of the screened individuals exhibit normal pressures or are mildly hypotensive

   **C.** It can be ascertained from the data that most of the individuals screened exhibit systolic hypertension

   **D.** The average diastolic blood pressure is approximately 80 mm Hg

   **E.** The average systolic blood pressure is approximately 120 mm Hg

**367.** A 62-year-old white man has a history of severe hypertension, two prior myocardial infarctions, and has a left ventricular ejection fraction of 15%. He presents with a 40-lb weight loss with a negative work-up for malignancy. From a cardiac standpoint, all of the following could explain this patient's weight loss **EXCEPT**

   **A.** digitalis intoxication

   **B.** protein loss in the gastrointestinal tract secondary to high right-sided pressure

   **C.** increased metabolic rate

   **D.** malabsorption of nutrients

   **E.** incomplete gastric emptying

**368.** A 36-year-old obese man with documented diastolic hypertension presents to your office. Which of the following is **LEAST** likely to help improve his diastolic hypertension?

   **A.** Decreased sodium intake

   **B.** Weight loss program

   **C.** Avoid excessive alcohol intake

   **D.** Decreased dietary fat intake

   **E.** Regular exercise program

**369.** You have recently discovered that a 71-year-old black woman has diabetes. With which symptom did she most likely present?

   **A.** Polydypsia

   **B.** Polyuria

   **C.** Dysuria

   **D.** Dizziness

   **E.** Vaginal itching

**370.** Increased risk of development of insulin dependent diabetes mellitus (IDDM) has been associated with all of the following **EXCEPT**
   **A.** being female
   **B.** being white
   **C.** changing seasons
   **D.** inheriting the HLA-DR3 gene
   **E.** inheriting the HLA-DR4 gene

**Questions 371–373:**
A 27-year-old female patient has had IDDM since age 7. During her routine office visit, she has the following vital signs: HR=72; RR=13; BP=140/90. Her HbA1C is 8.9.

**371.** This patient's primary risk for mortality from IDDM is
   **A.** renal disease
   **B.** ketoacidosis
   **C.** cardiovascular disease
   **D.** hypoglycemic coma
   **E.** stroke

**372.** The most common complication you would expect her to have is
   **A.** frequent urinary tract infections
   **B.** frequent yeast infections
   **C.** background retinopathy
   **D.** peripheral neuropathy
   **E.** angina

**373.** Interventions to prevent diabetic nephropathy in this patient could include all the following **EXCEPT**
   **A.** controlling blood pressure
   **B.** restricting protein intake
   **C.** increasing fluid intake
   **D.** intensifying glucose control
   **E.** close caloric control

**374.** Which *independent* risk factor would put a 60-year-old black woman with non–insulin dependent diabetes mellitus (NIDDM) at higher risk for cardiovascular disease?
**A.** Having a high LDL level
**B.** Having a high triglyceride level
**C.** Using oral hypoglycemics
**D.** Having a 20-year history of NIDDM
**E.** Being obese

**375.** You have just seen a 30-lb, 7-year-old boy with impetigo from a developing country village with poor sanitation. While at risk for many diseases, this child is at greatest risk for
**A.** Chagas' disease
**B.** glomerulonephritis
**C.** bacterial endocarditis
**D.** paralytic polio
**E.** hepatitis A

**376.** Which of the following groups do **NOT** have higher rates of renal disease than the American average?
**A.** Mexican-Americans
**B.** Asian-Americans
**C.** North American Indians
**D.** US blacks
**E.** Pacific Islanders

**377.** Both sensitive and specific tools are necessary for screening. When might serum creatinine **NOT** be a good screening tool?
**A.** In a muscular individual
**B.** In the young
**C.** In acute renal failure
**D.** When renal loss is <50%
**E.** High dietary protein

**378.** When a 10-year-old child with strep pharyngitis is treated with penicillin, which of the following is true?
**A.** Treatment will prevent the development of poststreptococcal glomerulonephritis (PSGN)
**B.** Treatment will reduce the risk of PSGN in contacts
**C.** Prophylactic treatment is recommended for his 3-year-old sister
**D.** Further evaluation should include repeated throat cultures
**E.** Contacts should be traced

**379.** A 42-year-old married woman presents with dysuria and increased urinary frequency. She also gives a complaint of frequent headaches, for which she takes Excedrin. The urine dipstick is positive for protein. Which of the following would most likely contribute to her dipstick results?
A. Urinary tract infection
B. Analgesic use
C. Dietary intake
D. Pregnancy
E. Dehydration

**Questions 380–382:**
Which of the following types of diabetes is *most closely* associated with the complication?

A. type I diabetes mellitus
B. type II diabetes mellitus
C. both type I and II diabetes

**380.** Nephropathy

**381.** The majority of diabetes end-stage renal diseases (ESRD) in the United States

**382.** Superimposed hypertension contributing to nephropathy

**383.** Hyaline membrane disease, or respiratory distress syndrome of the newborn (RDS) results from which deficiency?
A. Collagen type II
B. Collagen type I
C. Surfactant
D. Elastic fibers within the lungs
E. Mechanical deficits within the lungs

**384.** Which of the following is **NOT** a risk factor for RDS?
A. Prematurity
B. Perinatal asphyxia
C. Female sex
D. Cesarean section
E. Low gestational age

**385.** Which of the following is a common sequela of RDS?
   A. Bronchopulmonary dysplasia
   B. COPD
   C. Emphysema
   D. Asthma
   E. Pneumonia

**386.** Prenatal identification of fetuses at high risk for RDS can be accomplished by amniotic fluid analysis. Which are the ratios of phospholipids with the **LOWEST** risk for RDS?
   A. Sphingomyelin:lecithin 2:1
   B. Lecithin:sphingomyelin 2:1
   C. Sphingomyelin:lecithin 3:1
   D. Lecithin:sphingomyelin 1:1
   E. Lecithin:sphingomyelin 3:1

**387.** Which of the following treatment modalities have been shown to lessen the duration of mechanical ventilation and oxygen supplementation in newborns with RDS?
   A. Corticosteroids
   B. Nonsteroidal anti-inflammatory drugs
   C. Ultraviolet radiation
   D. Indocin
   E. Aspirin

**388.** Cystic fibrosis is a disorder primarily affecting which ethnic group?
   A. African-American
   B. Hispanic
   C. Asian
   D. White
   E. American Indian

**389.** Which of the following describes the genetic transmission of cystic fibrosis?
   A. Autosomal dominant
   B. X-linked recessive
   C. Autosomal recessive
   D. Autosomal dominant with variable penetration
   E. None of the above

**390.** Which of the following best describes the defect in cystic fibrosis?
   **A.** Epithelial cells oversecrete water into the mucus
   **B.** Inability of epithelial cells to secrete chloride ions
   **C.** Epithelial cells oversecrete sodium ions
   **D.** Inability of epithelial cells to produce protein
   **E.** Inability of the lung to clear secretions

**391.**

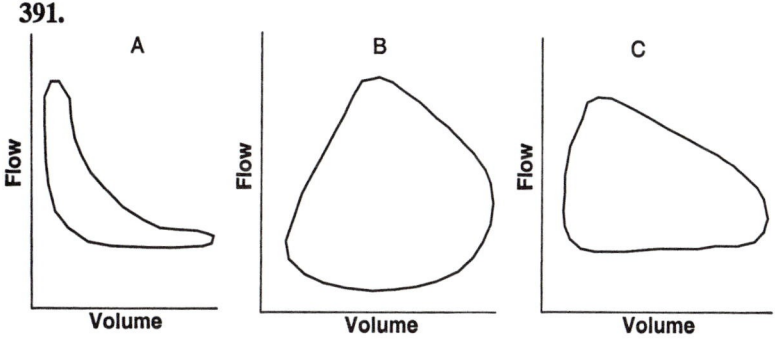

Which of the above flow volume curves best depicts COPD?
   **A.** Curve A
   **B.** Curve B
   **C.** Curve C
   **D.** None of the curves
   **E.** All could depict COPD

**392.** Which of the following organisms is associated with gastric and duodenal ulcers?
   **A.** *Streptococcus*
   **B.** *Entamoeba histolytic*
   **C.** *Helicobacter pylori*
   **D.** *Clostridium difficile*
   **E.** *Clostridium perfringens*

**393.** Which is a recommended treatment option for peptic ulcer?
   **A.** Amoxicillin and metronidazole
   **B.** Metronidazole alone
   **C.** Penicillin alone
   **D.** Vancomycin and metronidazole
   **E.** Any broad-spectrum antibiotic regimen is acceptable

**394.** Which of the following has been shown to double the mortality rate for peptic ulcers?
   A. Caffeine
   B. High-fat diet
   C. Alcohol
   D. Tobacco
   E. Age

**395.** Which of the following endogenous substances have been found to inhibit ulcer formation and promote healing?
   A. Adrenal steroids
   B. Estrogens
   C. Prostaglandin E
   D. Leukrotrienes
   E. Corticosteroids

**Questions 396–399:**
Choose the disease associated with the symptom or finding.

   A. ulcerative colitis
   B. Crohn's disease
   C. both
   D. neither

**396.** Rectal bleeding

**397.** Deep fissures and fistulas

**398.** Diffuse continuous involvement

**399.** Cobblestoning

**Questions 400–402:**
Name the disease associated with the finding.

   A. osteoarthritis
   B. rheumatoid arthritis
   C. both
   D. neither

**400.** Heberden's nodes

**401.** HLA-DR4

**402.** HLA-B27

**403.** An infant born at 4 lb 8 oz is at increased risk for cerebral palsy if any of the following conditions are present **EXCEPT**
A. severe asphyxia
B. maternal cigarette smoking during pregnancy
C. hyperbilirubinemia
D. intrauterine exposure to heavy metal
E. intrapartum physical injury

**404.** A 7-year-old black boy has an IQ of 60. The possible etiologic factors for his mild mental retardation include all of the following **EXCEPT**
A. sickle cell anemia
B. social deprivation
C. maternal short stature
D. maternal anemia
E. mother's nonverbal intelligence score

**405.** Isolated learning handicaps can be the only manifestation of which prenatal infection?
A. Cytomegalovirus
B. Herpes
C. Rubella
D. Syphilis
E. Gonorrhea

**406.** A 30-year-old white woman presents with chronic headaches. The psychologic characteristics associated with headache burden include all of the following **EXCEPT**
A. perfectionism
B. compulsion
C. inflexibility
D. depression
E. hypochondriasis

**407.** Persons with migraine headaches are at increased risk for
  A. stroke
  B. panic disorder
  C. myopia
  D. atherosclerotic heart disease
  E. psychoses

**408.** A 60-year-old woman has Parkinson's disease. She lives in the northeastern United States. Which other disease shows increased incidence in the northern hemisphere?
  A. Raynaud's disease
  B. Tay Sach's disease
  C. Alzheimer's disease
  D. Multiple sclerosis
  E. Rheumatoid arthritis

**409.** The most common surgical procedure in the United States is
  A. cholecystectomy
  B. tonsillectomy
  C. hysterectomy
  D. cataract extraction
  E. hernia repair

**410.** A 40-year-old computer operator presents with complaints of "eyestrain" and brow ache. Upon visual examination you would expect to find
  A. myopia
  B. hyperopia
  C. presbyopia
  D. emmetropia
  E. arteriovenous nicking

**411.** The major cause of blindness in the United States in persons over 50 years of age is
  A. age-related macular degeneration
  B. diabetes
  C. cataracts
  D. primary open-angle glaucoma
  E. trachoma

**Questions 412–415:**
In the general population there are relatively common co-occurrences of psychiatric disorders. Match the psychiatric disorders that often occur together (choose **ONE** correct answer; each answer can be used once, more than once, or not at all).

    **A.** alcoholism
    **B.** obsessive-compulsive disorder
    **C.** hypochondriasis
    **D.** somatization

**412.** Drug abuse

**413.** Panic disorder

**414.** Antisocial personality

**415.** Depression

**416.** A 40-year-old forklift operator presents with concerns about recent problems with memory and inability to concentrate. These problems are confirmed by his wife and by your examination. His problem is most likely which of the following?
    **A.** Alzheimer's disease
    **B.** Nicotine abuse
    **C.** Caffeine overdose
    **D.** Carbon monoxide toxicity
    **E.** Chronic alcoholism

**417.** A 7-year-old boy has been falling asleep in class every day. He claims to go to sleep each night around 9 PM and awaken at 7 AM. You suspect a sleep disorder. What is the most likely etiology of this disorder?
    **A.** Watching horror movies
    **B.** Hearing his parents argue constantly
    **C.** Drinking coke with dinner
    **D.** Having a new sibling in the house
    **E.** Poor nutrition

**418.** A 32-year-old woman presents with symptoms of depression. All of the following would make her more susceptible to depression **EXCEPT**
   A. not being employed outside the home
   B. having a poor relationship with her husband
   C. having three or more children under age six
   D. having lost a friend during childhood
   E. heavy use of sedatives

**419.** High rates of major depression have been reported for all of the following diseases **EXCEPT**
   A. thyroid disease
   B. multiple sclerosis
   C. Alzheimer's disease
   D. diabetes mellitus
   E. chronic pain

**420.** A 46-year-old white man is having trouble sleeping and difficulty concentrating. His social history reveals that he is a ditchdigger and often jumps when he hears cars roar by him. Which of the following pieces of historical information about this patient would most likely point to his diagnosis?
   A. He has hearing loss in the high frequencies
   B. He fought in the Vietnam war
   C. He works a second job as a security guard
   D. He has one glass of scotch per day
   E. He is divorced

**421.** Because medical care is becoming increasingly effective, it is prolonging the lives of many mentally retarded persons. In addition, new scientific technology and improved methods of prevention offer the prospect of eliminating a number of specific medical disorders altogether. Based on these assertions, which of the following conclusions can be drawn?
   A. Prevention reduces the incidence of mental retardation, and medical care decreases the prevalence
   B. Prevention reduces the incidence of mental retardation, and medical care increases the prevalence
   C. Both prevention and medical care increase the incidence of mental retardation

    **D.** Both prevention and medical care reduce the incidence of mental retardation

    **E.** None of the above

**422.** When describing mental retardation, the term referring to an underlying biologic disorder is

    **A.** disability

    **B.** handicap

    **C.** impairment

    **D.** deficiency

    **E.** all are interchangeable

**423.** Given that IQ tests are constructed to produce a mean score of 100 and a standard deviation of 15 among the population at large, what percentage of the population will be expected to score below 70?

    **A.** 7.5%

    **B.** 5.5%

    **C.** 3.5%

    **D.** 2.5%

    **E.** 1.5%

**424.**        **Prevalence of Mental Retardation:**

| Location | Age | Rate per 1000 |
| --- | --- | --- |
| Oregon | 12–14 | 25.0 |
| England | 9–14 | 35.0 |
| California | 8–10 | 55.0 |
| Scotland | 9–14 | 37.0 |

Based on the above information, which of the following best exemplifies the prediction about the prevalence of mental retardation calculated in Question 423?

    **A.** The Oregon group

    **B.** The England group

    **C.** The California group

    **D.** The Scotland group

    **E.** None

**425.** For autosomal recessive disorders such as phenylketonuria, which of the following is true?
   **A.** For a female child to be affected, the father must be affected
   **B.** Male offspring of female carriers have a 50% chance of being affected
   **C.** Both parents are unaffected carriers
   **D.** One parent is an unaffected carrier
   **E.** One parent must be an affected carrier

**426.** A newborn infant is noted to have low birth weight, narrow palpebral fissures, microcephaly, and flattened nasolabial facies. Which of the following is the most likely substance the mother was exposed to prenatally?
   **A.** Lead
   **B.** Mercury
   **C.** Alcohol
   **D.** Benzene
   **E.** Carbon monoxide

**427.** Infectious agents that can cause congenital defects following prenatal infection include all of the following **EXCEPT**
   **A.** syphilis
   **B.** rubella
   **C.** cytomegalovirus
   **D.** gonorrhea
   **E.** toxoplasmosis

**428.** A teenage mother on welfare lives in a local housing project. She states her 8-year-old child has recently been nauseated with vomiting and is exhibiting poor concentration and possible seizures. Which of the following is the most likely cause?
   **A.** The presence of peeling paint on any buildings
   **B.** The source of water
   **C.** The presence of asbestos in the ceilings
   **D.** Any recent outbreaks of pertussis in the neighborhood
   **E.** Food-borne bacteria

**429.** A "nervous" disorder first described in India led to central nervous system dysfunction, cerebral palsy, and mental retardation. A similar disorder was seen as a result of congenital hypothyroidism. Which of the following was likely to be deficient in the diet?
   **A.** Sodium
   **B.** Zinc
   **C.** Iodine
   **D.** Potassium
   **E.** Chloride

**430.** Of the following activities of daily living (ADL) among the elderly, which are the most common dependencies?
   **A.** Eating
   **B.** Toileting
   **C.** Bathing
   **D.** Incontinence
   **E.** Shopping

**431.** Which of the following medical conditions is most strongly associated with ADL limitations?
   **A.** Hip fracture
   **B.** Myocardial infarction
   **C.** Emphysema
   **D.** Transient ischemic attack
   **E.** COPD

**432.** One forecast regarding anticipated societal burdens of the elderly is known as the "compression of morbidity" thesis. This thesis maintains that chronic disease and disability are being postponed or prevented as a result of risk-reducing and health-promoting measures. If this thesis is correct, which of the following conclusions can be drawn?
   **A.** Future prevalence rates of disability and chronic care will increase
   **B.** Future prevalence rates of disability and chronic care will diminish
   **C.** Future prevalence rates of disability and chronic care will remain unchanged
   **D.** The prevalence of disability will not affect health care costs
   **E.** No conclusions can be validly drawn

**433.** Another forecast regarding anticipated societal burdens is known as the "failure of success" thesis. This thesis argues that prolongation of life expectancy among the elderly is due to advances in technology that prolong the duration of certain chronic disabling conditions. If this thesis is correct, which of the following conclusions can be drawn?
  **A.** Future prevalence rates of disability and chronic care will increase relative to current rates
  **B.** Future prevalence rates of disability and chronic care will decrease relative to current rates
  **C.** Future prevalence rates of disability and chronic care will remain unchanged
  **D.** No conclusions can be validly drawn
  **E.** The prevalence of disability will not affect health care costs

**434.** Which of the following is **NOT** an intrinsic biologic consequence of aging?
  **A.** Decrease in bone density
  **B.** Modification of lens protein leading to loss of vision
  **C.** Stiffening of arterial walls
  **D.** Increase in maximum oxygen consumption
  **E.** Limitation of joint flexibility

**435.** A 72-year-old widowed woman sustained a fracture to her right hip 3 months ago. Which of the following is most likely to provide a substantial positive impact on this patient's health?
  **A.** Reduction in dietary fat and cholesterol intake
  **B.** Weight reduction
  **C.** Estrogen replacement therapy
  **D.** Visual acuity examinations
  **E.** Removal of throw rugs

**Questions 436–438:**
A 65-year-old woman presents complaining of inadvertent loss of urine occurring intermittently over the past several weeks. She denies prior abdominal or pelvic surgery. She does admit to recent dysuria and mild hematuria.

**436.** Which of the following is the most likely diagnosis?
  **A.** Stress incontinence
  **B.** Overflow incontinence

    **C.** Functional incontinence
    **D.** Urge incontinence
    **E.** None of the above

**437.** Which of the following would be most helpful in making a diagnosis?
    **A.** Ultrasound
    **B.** CBC
    **C.** Urinalysis
    **D.** Pelvic examination
    **E.** Cervical cultures

**438.** If a urinary tract infection were suspected and appropriate antibiotic therapy failed to alleviate the symptoms, what would be the next choice of therapy?
    **A.** Anticholinergic agents
    **B.** A different class of antibiotic
    **C.** Surgical intervention
    **D.** Intermittent catheter drainage
    **E.** Psychologic counseling

**Questions 439–442:**
A 78-year-old man exhibits shuffling gait, tremulous hands with "pill-rolling" movements, generalized cognitive impairment, and has fallen twice in the past month.

**439.** Which of the following is highest on the differential diagnosis list?
    **A.** Alzheimer's disease
    **B.** Multi-infarct dementia
    **C.** Parkinson's disease
    **D.** Cerebrovascular disease
    **E.** Guillain-Barré syndrome

**440.** What best describes the neurotransmitter associated with this condition?
    **A.** Deficiency of GABA
    **B.** Excess of GABA
    **C.** Excess of dopamine
    **D.** Deficiency of dopamine
    **E.** Deficiency of serotonin

**441.** Which of the following medications should be discontinued in this patient?
A. Labetalol
B. Haldol
C. Propranolol
D. Diphenhydramine
E. Captopril

**442.** Which of the following treatment options, in addition to pharmacologic agents, will be most beneficial?
A. Physical therapy
B. Dietary modification
C. Psychologic counseling
D. Surgical consultation
E. Exercise program

**443.** The recommended daily allowances (RDAs) are based on age, body size, gender, and developmental stage and make recommendations for all of the following **EXCEPT**
A. several vitamins
B. protein
C. some minerals
D. fiber
E. other nutrients

**444.** Recommended daily allowances in the United States are designed to
A. give the minimum daily requirement of minerals and vitamins
B. prevent deficiencies
C. give exact recommendations for nutritional requirements
D. establish specific energy need for individuals
E. guide the food production industry

**445.** A 72-year-old male patient presents with seborrheic skin lesions about the eyes, nose, and mouth. He has a 12-year history of drinking two glasses of vodka per day. He has recently started on INH. This patient's problem is
A. pyridoxine deficiency
B. INH toxicity
C. retin A toxicity
D. thiamine deficiency
E. drug-induced hepatitis

**446.** The major contributing cause of death among young children in developing countries is
   **A.** lack of immunizations
   **B.** diarrhea
   **C.** respiratory infections
   **D.** malnutrition
   **E.** malaria

**447.** A 1-1/2-year-old Native American boy is brought to you because his mother is concerned over his carious teeth. You should advise her to do which of the following?
   **A.** See a dentist
   **B.** Stop giving him a bottle
   **C.** Stop giving him a pacifier
   **D.** Brush his teeth
   **E.** Wait until his permanent teeth emerge

**448.** The fluoride in a community's water supply is 0.5 ppm. You would recommend which of the following for a 2-1/2-year-old child?
   **A.** Supplement with 0.25 mg/d of fluoride
   **B.** Supplement with 0.50 mg/d of fluoride
   **C.** Supplement with 1.0 mg/d of fluoride
   **D.** Do not supplement with fluoride
   **E.** Use bottled water

**449.** Prevention of periodontal disease includes all of the following **EXCEPT**
   **A.** rinsing one's mouth with Listerine or Peridex
   **B.** brushing one's teeth
   **C.** flossing one's teeth
   **D.** taking 800 mg of calcium daily
   **E.** avoiding tobacco use

**450.** The leading cause of potential years of life lost is
   **A.** unintentional injury
   **B.** SIDS
   **C.** HIV and AIDS
   **D.** cancer
   **E.** cardiovascular disease

**451.** The victim of those who commit a homicide while under the influence of alcohol and drugs is **LEAST** likely to be a
  A. friend
  B. child
  C. spouse
  D. stranger
  E. parent

**452.** A 30-year-old white woman presents with complaints of chest pain. On examination you find ecchymosis on her chest and abdomen. She denies any injury. This woman is at risk for all the following sequelae of this syndrome **EXCEPT**
  A. panic disorder
  B. attempted suicide
  C. rape
  D. psychotic break
  E. alcoholism

**453.** Many children who witness violence suffer **SPECIFICALLY** from
  A. bed-wetting
  B. nightmares
  C. anxiety
  D. post-traumatic stress disorder
  E. poor eating habits

**454.** A 15-year-old girl commits suicide. Her method was most likely
  A. wrist slitting
  B. overdosing
  C. hanging
  D. shooting
  E. automobile accident

**455.** You diagnose a 3-year-old child with battered child syndrome. This child is at risk for all of the following **EXCEPT**
  A. mild mental retardation
  B. low performance on standardized tests of intelligence
  C. a propensity to aggression in adolescence
  D. a language disorder
  E. sleeping and eating changes

**456.** With regard to mortality in relation to smoking, which is **IN-CORRECT?**
  **A.** Current male cigarette smokers have a 70% greater chance of dying from disease than nonsmokers
  **B.** Specific mortality rates are directly proportional to the amount smoked and the years of cigarette smoking
  **C.** Specific mortality rates are higher for those who initiated their smoking at younger ages
  **D.** Former cigarette smokers carry their increased mortality rate with them after they stop smoking
  **E.** Fifteen years after cessation, mortality rates of former smokers approach that of those who have never smoked

**457.** Which is the **INCORRECT** statement with regard to smoking and cancer of the lungs?
  **A.** The most definite causal relationship between the use of tobacco and any disease is with lung cancer
  **B.** Lung cancer mortality rates in women are increasing much more slowly than in men
  **C.** Cancer of the lungs has become the leading cause of cancer deaths in women in the 1990s
  **D.** The use of filter cigarettes with low tar and nicotine content decreases lung cancer mortality
  **E.** Smokers experience decrease in lung cancer mortality rates, which approaches the rate of nonsmokers, after 10 or 15 years of cessation

**458.** Which of the following is the most expensive occupational health problem?
  **A.** Circulatory diseases
  **B.** Bone and joint disorder
  **C.** Digestive disorders
  **D.** Allergic disorders
  **E.** Upper respiratory infections

**459.** The leading cause of fatal home accidents is
  **A.** fires
  **B.** explosions
  **C.** poisoning
  **D.** falls
  **E.** firearms

**460.** Increased frequency of injuries are associated with all of the following **EXCEPT**
   A. male sex
   B. age 25 to 40
   C. blacks
   D. Native Americans
   E. elderly

**461.** What is the largest cause of unintentional injury deaths in the United States?
   A. Motor vehicle accidents
   B. Gun-shot wounds
   C. Industrial accidents
   D. Falls
   E. Climatic disasters

**462.** The most frequent cause of house fires is
   A. faulty electrical wiring
   B. dropped cigarettes
   C. children playing with matches
   D. gas leaks
   E. barbecues

**463.** Concerning infant mortality in the United States, which is the **INCORRECT** statement?
   A. Gastroenteritis is a rare cause of infant death in the United States today
   B. The infant mortality rate in the United States is lower than that found in Sweden and the Netherlands
   C. Infant mortality rates show large differences between races in the United States
   D. High infant and maternal mortality rates occur among teenage mothers, especially the very young ones
   E. Recent infant mortality rates (since 1975) run around 16/1000 live births, down from about 30/1000 in 1950

**464.** How did accidents rank in 1987 as a cause of overall death in the United States?
   A. Second
   B. Third

    **C.** Fourth
    **D.** Fifth
    **E.** Seventh

**465.** Accidents are the leading cause of death for ages
    **A.** 1 to 21
    **B.** 1 to 38
    **C.** 1 to 54
    **D.** 3 to 24
    **E.** 9 to 45

**466.** The leading cause of years of potential life lost for people under age 65 in the United States for 1987 is
    **A.** heart disease
    **B.** cancer
    **C.** stroke
    **D.** unintentional injuries
    **E.** pulmonary disease

**467.** The 1976–1986 trend in accidental death rates in the United States for all causes was
    **A.** relatively unchanged for all age groups
    **B.** downward for all age groups
    **C.** upward for all age groups
    **D.** downward for ages under 5 years to 25 to 44, but upward 45 and over
    **E.** upward for ages under 5 years to 25 to 44, but downward 45 and over

**468.** The most common reason given by those who oppose mandatory seat belt use laws is
    **A.** such laws infringe on personal liberty
    **B.** such laws are not effective in saving lives
    **C.** the enforcement cost of such laws is too high
    **D.** there are too many mechanical failures, making 100% seat belt use impractical
    **E.** interference with survival of the fittest principle

**469.** Which of the following is **NOT** true?
- **A.** All states require children to use restraining devices in automobiles
- **B.** The public is more favorable toward laws requiring the use of child restraint devices than mandatory seat belt laws for adults
- **C.** There is no association between the use of seat belts by adults and compliance with laws requiring the use of child restraint devices
- **D.** Studies show that the use of child restraint devices saves lives
- **E.** Public acceptance is so high that it seems unlikely that any state will try to repeal laws requiring the use of child restraint devices in autos

**470.** The proportion of fatal motor vehicle accidents in which drinking alcoholic beverages is a factor is
- **A.** 15% to 20%
- **B.** 25% to 35%
- **C.** 40% to 45%
- **D.** 50% to 55%
- **E.** 65% to 70%

**471.** A fatal traffic crash is considered alcohol-related by the National Highway Traffic Safety Administration (NHTSA) if either a driver or nonoccupant (eg, a pedestrian) had a blood alcohol concentration (BAC) of
- **A.** a detectable level
- **B.** 0.01 g/dL
- **C.** 0.05 g/dL
- **D.** 0.08 g/dL
- **E.** 1.00 g/dL

**472.** The type of vehicle with the highest proportion of involvement in fatal accidents is
- **A.** passenger car
- **B.** truck, truck tractor, or truck tractor semitrailer
- **C.** motorcycle, motor scooter, motorbike
- **D.** taxicab
- **E.** commercial bus

**473.** The category in which the most disabling injuries occurred in 1986 was
  A. motor vehicle accidents
  B. work accidents
  C. public accidents
  D. home accidents
  E. other

**474.** The most dangerous area of work-related accidents in terms of fatalities is
  A. agriculture (includes forestry and fishing)
  B. mining, quarrying
  C. construction
  D. transportation and public utilities
  E. manufacturing

**475.** Concerning cancer morbidity and mortality, which is the **INCORRECT** statement?
  A. A child born in the United States in 1985 had more than a one in three chance of eventually developing an invasive cancer
  B. For white women the probability of developing cancer of the breast during their lifetime is about 1 in 10
  C. Currently it is projected that the chances of developing any form of cancer is greater for men than for women
  D. The incidence of cancer of the prostate in men has overtaken lung cancer
  E. In men at age 65 the probability of lung cancer increases and prostate cancer decreases, especially in blacks

# Noncommunicable and Chronic Diseases

## Answers and Discussion

**326.** **(C)** Chronic diseases and conditions such as cancer, diseases of the cardiovascular system, cirrhosis, and chronic respiratory diseases are associated with a particular behavior and thus can probably be treated or prevented with lifestyle change. Tuberculosis is an infectious disease primarily influenced by environmental factors. (**Ref. 2,** pp. 687, 688)

**327.** **(D)** People who are not married have higher mortality rates than married people. Divorced single white men have higher mortality rates for virtually every major cause of death (except leukemia for divorced men and genital cancer for single men). Similarly, divorced and single white women, compared with those who are married, have higher death rates for almost all causes of death. (**Ref. 2,** p. 690)

**328.** **(B)** People in the lowest socioeconomic level have the highest rates of morbidity and mortality. Various studies have shown that people who changed jobs or residencies frequently had higher rates of disease. Studies have shown that persons with social support have lower morbidity and mortality rates than those who do not. One of the most well-established facts among students of health and disease is that men have higher mortality rates than women. (**Ref. 2,** pp. 688–693)

**329.** **(C)** Behavioral risk factors have become increasingly visible as underlying causes of preventable morbidity and premature death. Researchers undertook to measure underlying risk factors that contribute to 14 leading causes of morbidity and mortality. They identified alcohol abuse, tobacco use, unintentional injury, and unintended pregnancy as the highest priority risk factors. Four other risk factors that ranked nearly as high were obesity and high serum cholesterol levels, handguns, and dental problems. **(Ref. 2, p. 701)**

**330.** **(C)** All contribute to significant cancer deaths, but smoking has the greatest impact on total cancer mortality. **(Ref. 2, pp. 701, 702)**

**331.** **(B)** Smoking has been estimated to cause 30% of the life years lost from cardiovascular disease; 18% of life years lost was attributed to high blood pressure and 9% to elevated serum cholesterol. **(Ref. 2, p. 701)**

**332.** **(A)** Combined results of multiple epidemiologic studies show that smokers average a twofold increased risk of a myocardial infarction, a tenfold increased risk for lung cancer, and a sixfold increased risk for COPD. Risk for bladder and kidney cancer are increased less than twofold. **(Ref. 2, p. 715)**

**333.** **(B)** While all are risk factors for cardiovascular disease, smoking is the most significant contributor to peripheral vascular disease. **(Ref. 2, p. 719)**

**334.** **(D)** Smoking is estimated to cause 45% and 41%, respectively, of all CHD deaths of men and women less than 65 years of age, with 21% and 12% being the corresponding percentages for men and women 65 years of age and older. On the basis of results from a variety of sources, a reasonable estimate is that 30% to 40% of all CHD deaths are attributable to smoking. **(Ref. 2, p. 716)**

**335.** **(E)** The CDC definition for the fetal tobacco syndrome includes **A** through **D**. The placental:birth weight ratio is larger than normal to provide adequate fetal oxygenation. **(Ref. 2, p. 725)**

**336.** **(E)** Carcinoma of the mouth, larynx, pharynx, esophagus, liver, lung; alcoholic cardiomyopathy; other cardiovascular disease; pneumonia; peptic ulcers; liver cirrhosis; suicide; and accidents are all associated with the excess mortality of chronic heavy drinkers. Tuberculosis is associated with variables such as heavy tobacco smoking, poor food habits, other personal neglect, and increased environmental hazards. (**Ref. 2,** p. 743)

**337. (D)** (**Ref. 2,** p. 746)

**338. (E)** North America, Australia and New Zealand, and Europe are the most economically developed regions. They also share similar cultural heritages and have a long history of acceptance and use of alcohol. (**Ref. 2,** p. 745)

**339. (B)** Rules and regulations implementing the Alcoholic Beverage Act require the warnings on labels of all containers of alcoholic beverages bottled on or after November 18, 1989. (**Ref. 2,** p. 757)

**340. (C)** Adolescents make up the largest segment of our population that abuses drugs. Homicides, suicides, and accidents account for over 77% of adolescent deaths, and drug abuse is implicated in over half of these deaths. (**Ref. 2,** p. 769)

**341. (C)** Narcotics withdrawal syndrome causes watery eyes, runny nose, yawning, loss of appetite, irritability, tremors, panic, cramps, nausea, chills, and sweating; withdrawal symptoms from depressants include anxiety, insomnia, tremors, delirium, convulsions, and possible death; withdrawal symptoms from stimulants include, apathy, long periods of sleep, irritability, depression and disorientation; withdrawal symptoms from cannabis include insomnia, hyperactivity, and decreased appetite occasionally reported. There has been no withdrawal syndrome reported for hallucinogens. (**Ref. 2,** pp. 770–772)

**342. (D)** The following risk factors have been identified relatively consistently in the initiation or augmentation of drug abuse in adolescents and young adults: parents' drug use, family strife, early alcohol use, low socio–economic status, poor school grades, depression, age, parents' educational level, peer drug use, sensation seeking, deviance, low self-esteem, aggression. Two factors that are associated with declines in drug use in young adults are employment and marriage. (**Ref. 2,** p. 778)

**343. (A)** These studies have shown that sons of alcoholic mothers or fathers are at increased risk for alcoholism compared with the general population. For daughters, a biological mother with alcoholism significantly increased the rate of alcoholism. Rates for women with an alcoholic biological father were not significantly higher than those found in women whose biological parents were not alcoholics. **(Ref. 2,** p. 777)

**344. (C)** The purpose of a screening test is to detect individuals with risk factors that predispose to disease development or with asymptomatic diseases that can be effectively treated. **(Ref. 2,** p. 807)

**345. (D)** Sensitivity is the proportional detection of individuals with the disease of interest in the tested population.

$$\text{Sensitivity} = \frac{\text{true positives}}{\text{true positives and false negatives}} \times 100$$

**(Ref. 2,** p. 807)

**346. (A)** Specificity is the proportional detection of individuals *without* the disease of interest.

$$\text{Sensitivity} = \frac{\text{true negatives}}{\text{true negatives and false positives}} \times 100$$

**(Ref. 2,** p. 807)

**347. (B)** The predictive value of a positive test is the proportion of all individuals with positive tests who have the disease.

$$\text{Positive predictive value} = \frac{\text{true positives}}{\text{true positives and false positives}} \times 100$$

**(Ref. 2,** p. 807)

**348. (C)** The predictive value of a negative test is the proportion of all individuals with negative tests who are nondiseased.

$$\text{Negative predictive value} = \frac{\text{true negatives}}{\text{true negatives and false negatives}} \times 100$$

**(Ref. 2,** p. 807)

**349. (A)** The receiver operating characteristic curve displays the true positive ratio on the ordinate and the false positive ratio on the abscissa. Curve A demonstrates the greatest true positive ratio or sensitivity at all points. (**Ref. 2,** pp. 807, 808)

**350. (E)** The specificity or false positive ratio is exhibited on the abscissa. Curve E demonstrates the greatest false positive ratio at each point along the ordinate. (**Ref. 2,** pp. 807, 808)

**351. (C)** In the United States the 1982–1986 cancer rates for men in decreasing order are: prostate (85%), lung (84%), colon (42%), bladder (28%), rectum (19%). (**Ref. 2,** pp. 811, 812)

**352. (A)** In the United States the 1982–1986 cancer rates for women in decreasing order are: breast (97%), lung (34%), colon (32%), uterus (22%), ovary (14%). (**Ref. 2,** pp. 811, 812)

**353. (A)** Cancers of the colon are thought to be related to diets rich in animal fat and are linked to a "western" type of lifestyle. (**Ref. 2,** p. 813)

**354. (A)** Cancers of the rectum are thought to be related to diets rich in animal fat and are linked to a "western" type of lifestyle. (**Ref. 2,** p. 813)

**355. (D)** Lung and laryngeal cancer are related to chemical irritants, most commonly to smoking. In men in the United States, tobacco is responsible for approximately 90% of all cases of lung cancer. (**Ref. 2,** pp. 813, 816)

**356. (B)** Stomach cancer has been linked to the use of preserved foods. (**Ref. 2,** p. 813)

**357. (E)** Nasopharyngeal cancer is thought to be related to Epstein-Barr virus. Nearly 100% of these patients have antibodies against EBV compared with much lower percentages in controls. (**Ref. 2,** pp. 813, 819)

**358. (C)** Hepatocellular carcinoma is directly related to infection with hepatitis B virus. The disease appears to develop in individuals who become chronic carriers of the hepatitis B surface antigen. (**Ref. 2,** pp. 813, 819)

**359. (G)** The epidemiologic features of cervical cancer suggest strongly that one or more types of sexually transmitted diseases play a role in their development. The most frequently associated sexually transmitted disease is human papilloma virus. HPV types 16 and 18 are found most commonly with invasive cancers, whereas types 6 and 11 are less aggressive. (**Ref. 2,** pp. 813, 819, 820)

**360. (D)** Unstable angina pectoris involves rest angina that is usually prolonged, and the onset of angina has occurred within 2 months of the initial presentation. The pain increases in intensity, duration, and frequency. Chronic stable angina episodes are typically caused by exertion, usually last less than 5 minutes, and are relieved by rest. Prinzmetal's angina occurs during rest or awakens the patient from sleep. It may be accompanied by palpitations or severe shortness of breath, is explosive in onset, and severe in nature. Silent ischemia is asymptomatic. (**Ref. 2,** p. 832; **Ref. 22,** pp. 1077–1085)

**361. (A)** A patient with unstable angina should be admitted promptly to the hospital for observation, further diagnosis, and treatment. When unstable angina is accompanied with ECG changes consistent with ischemia, it is almost always associated with critical stenosis in one or more major coronary arteries. (**Ref. 22,** pp. 1083, 1084)

**362. (A)** Symptoms are highly suggestive of a group A streptococcal infection with several of the minor Jones criteria for rheumatic fever, such as fever and arthralgia. A throat culture for group A strep is warranted. (**Ref. 2,** pp. 153, 840)

**363. (D)** Treatment of choice for group A streptococcal infections causing rheumatic fever is penicillin. (**Ref. 2,** p. 841)

**364. (C)** Acute glomerulonephritis may follow a group A streptococcal infection and is manifested by hematuria, proteinuria, and RBC casts. (**Ref. 2,** p. 155)

**365. (C)** The modal value is the most frequently occurring value, which is 80 to 90 for this population. (**Ref. 2,** pp. 849, 850)

**366. (A)** The data are skewed to the right with a majority exhibiting elevated diastolic blood pressures in the moderate to severe levels.

An average cannot be computed on this data set because it is a skewed distribution. (**Ref. 2,** pp. 849, 850)

**367.** **(E)** With severe chronic heart failure, severe weight loss can be caused by a number of factors. Elevation of the metabolic rate resulting from increased respiratory muscle work is a cause. Impaired intestinal absorption resulting from venous congestion and protein losing enteropathies are other causes. Digitalis toxicity can cause anorexia, nausea, and vomiting. Congestive hepatomegaly and abdominal fullness can lead to ascites and impaired gastric filling and early satiety. (**Ref. 83,** pp. 49, 64)

**368.** **(A)** Within populations, salt intake and urinary sodium excretion were positively correlated with systolic pressure more often than with diastolic pressure. It is generally advised that weight loss, low dietary fat intake, and avoidance of excessive alcohol intake will benefit all hypertensives. (**Ref. 2,** pp. 852–854)

**369.** **(C)** The diagnosis of non–insulin-dependent diabetes mellitus (NIDDM) is often made when a patient presents with a complication of the disease rather than classical symptoms of diabetes. The patient presented with a urinary tract infection, but her urine dipstick showed positive for albumin, indicating the presence of microvascular disease of the kidney secondary to diabetes. (**Ref. 2,** pp. 873, 874)

**370.** **(A)** For IDDM the overall incidence rates of males and females is about the same. The incidence for whites is about 1.5 times that of blacks. Most IDDM patients possess either the HLA-DR3 or HLA-DR4 allele or both. Infections associated with changing seasons may contribute to the condition. (**Ref. 2,** p. 876)

**371.** **(A)** This patient is in her second decade of IDDM during which time renal disease becomes the major cause of death. During the first decade, the primary cause of death is ketoacidosis and after the second decade it is renal and cardiovascular disease. (**Ref. 2,** p. 878)

**372.** **(C)** Approximately 80% to 90% of patients with IDDM have some evidence of background retinopathy after having IDDM for at least 20 years. (**Ref. 2,** p. 878)

**373. (C)** Treatment of hypertension (or mildly elevated blood pressure), protein restriction, and intensified glucose control may reduce albuminuria in the early stages. **(Ref. 2, p. 879)**

**374. (B)** Triglyceride level is an independent risk factor for cardiovascular disease in diabetes. The others are probably not *independent* of NIDDM and diabetes, though they are risk factors for cardiovascular disease. **(Ref. 2, p. 879)**

**375. (B)** Glomerulonephritis is the most common cause of renal failure and renal death in the developing world. Susceptibility is enhanced by infections, malnutrition, and poor living conditions. Rates fall as these conditions improve. He has probably already had both hepatitis A and polio and developed immunity. **(Ref. 2, p. 861)**

**376. (B)** In western societies, US blacks, North American Indians, Hispanics, and Mexican-Americans, urban South African blacks, and Pacific Islanders have especially high rates of renal disease, in part from hypertension and diabetes. **(Ref. 2, p. 859)**

**377. (D)** Serum creatinine provides an approximate measure of renal insufficiency. In cases of muscle leanness, diets low in protein, old age, renal loss <50%, and progressive loss of renal function in severe renal failure, creatinine levels may not reflect the true state of renal function. **(Ref. 2, p. 859)**

**378. (B)** Antibiotic treatment does not prevent poststreptococcal glomerulonephritis (PSGN) in a person with streptococcal infection. Antibiotic treatment may reduce the antistreptolysin O (ASO) antibody titer. Only certain strains of streptococci, including nontypeable group A strep, have nephritogenic potential. Even infection with nephritogenic strains, however, results in glomerulonephritis only in about 15% of infections. Antibiotic treatment does reduce the chance of spread to others and of subsequent PSGN in contacts. Prophylactic treatment is only recommended during epidemics and for siblings or families of patients with known PSGN. **(Ref. 2, p. 862)**

**379. (B)** Analgesic nephropathy (AN) mainly afflicts middle-aged women. Minimal cumulative ingestion of at least 3 to 5 kg of analgesic mixtures can cause AN. Caffeine intake, dehydration, and certain trace elements in water might facilitate renal injury. Urinary tract infections (UTI) have dipstick findings of leukocytes, not protein. UTIs rarely lead to renal damage unless associated with diabetes, pregnancy, reflux, obstruction, or neurogenic bladder. (**Ref. 2,** p. 865)

**380.** **(C)** Diabetic nephropathy can occur in both type I and type II diabetics. It is a leading cause of kidney failure in the western world. (**Ref. 2,** p. 860)

**381.** **(B)** Type II diabetes accounts for the majority of diabetic end-stage renal disease (ESRD) in the United States. (**Ref. 2,** p. 860)

**382.** **(A)** Coexisting hypertension or high normal blood pressures are powerful risk factors for nephropathy in type I diabetes. (**Ref. 2,** p. 861)

**383.** **(C)** RDS is the result of surfactant deficiency. (**Ref. 2,** p. 885)

**384.** **(C)** Risk factors for RDS include prematurity, perinatal asphyxia, male sex, cesarean section, low gestational age. (**Ref. 2,** p. 885)

**385.** **(A)** Bronchopulmonary dysplasia occurs as a frequent sequela of RDS characterized by persistent pulmonary dysfunction and oxygen dependence after 1 month of age. (**Ref. 2,** p. 885)

**386.** **(B)** Prenatal identification of RDS by amniotic fluid analysis shows the lowest risk associated with a lecithin:sphingomyelin ratio of 2:1. (**Ref. 2,** p. 886)

**387.** **(A)** Corticosteroids have been shown to lessen the duration of treatment for RDS. (**Ref. 2,** p. 886)

**388.** **(D)** Cystic fibrosis occurs in 1/2000 live births in the United States, most commonly affecting the white population (5%). (**Ref. 2,** p. 886)

**389.** **(C)** Cystic fibrosis is an autosomal recessive disorder. (**Ref. 2,** p. 886)

**390. (B)** The defect in cystic fibrosis concerns the epithelial cells' inability to secrete chloride ions. (**Ref. 2,** p. 886)

**391. (A)** Curve A demonstrates obstructive lung disease; curve B is normal; curve C depicts reactive airway disease. (**Ref. 2,** p. 890)

**392. (C)** *Helicobacter pylori* is the bacterium associated with gastric and duodenal ulcers. (**Ref. 2,** p. 897)

**393. (A)** Amoxicillin and metronidazole together are the recommended regimen. (**Ref. 82,** pp. 65–69)

**394. (D)** Cigarette smoking has been shown to double the mortality rate for peptic ulcer disease. Caffeine and alcohol are not significant risk factors. (**Ref. 2,** p. 809)

**395. (C)** Prostaglandin E, especially $E_2$, has been shown to produce an antisecretory effect on parietal cells and inhibit gastric acid secretion. (**Ref. 2,** p. 901)

**396. (C); 397. (B); 398. (A); 399. (B)** Both Crohn's disease and ulcerative colitis can produce rectal bleeding. Crohn's disease produces deep fissures and fistulas with cobblestoning; ulcerative colitis produces diffuse continuous involvement of the gastrointestinal tract. (**Ref. 77,** p. 292)

**400. (A); 401. (B); 402. (D)** Osteoarthritis involves joint swelling, morning stiffness, and Heberden's nodes. Rheumatoid arthritis is associated with HLA-DR4. Ankylosing spondylitis is associated with HLA-B27. (**Ref. 2,** pp. 917–919)

**403. (B)** The incidence of cerebral palsy is estimated at 2.5 cases per 1000 live births. Maternal smoking is not a risk factor for cerebral palsy. Potential causes of cerebral palsy include intrapartum and postnatal conditions, such as intrauterine exposure to heavy metals, neonatal hyperbilirubinemia, and severe asphyxia. (**Ref. 2,** pp. 929, 930)

**404. (A)** Blacks have a higher rate of mild mental retardation than whites. Risk factors for mild mental retardation include social deprivation, mother's nonverbal intelligence score, maternal short stature, maternal late age of menarche, and complications of pregnancy, such as urinary tract infection, anemia, and toxemia. (**Ref. 2,** p. 930)

**405. (C)** Prenatal rubella infection is the only prenatal infection capable of damaging the brain that has been linked to isolated learning handicaps. (**Ref. 2,** p. 931)

**406. (B)** Psychosocial characteristics associated with headache burden, especially migraine, include perfectionism, inflexibility, hypochondriasis, anxiety, and depression. (**Ref. 2,** p. 932)

**407. (D)** Persons with migraines appear to be at greater risk of hypertension and atherosclerotic heart disease. (**Ref. 2,** p. 932)

**408. (D)** The prevalence of multiple sclerosis is highest in the northern hemisphere, increasing as latitude increases. Studies have shown that children who migrate from areas of high prevalence to areas of low prevalence take on the risk level of their new environment. Mortality rates from Parkinson's disease are also higher in the northern hemisphere as compared with the southern. (**Ref. 2,** pp. 932, 933)

**409. (D)** Cataract extraction is the most common major surgical procedure in the United States. (**Ref. 2,** p. 937)

**410. (B)** Hyperopia is farsightedness. It is the most common refractive error. It often goes unrecognized until middle age, when accommodation declines and the patient experiences brow ache, asthenopia (fatigue), or both. Myopia is nearsightedness. Presbyopia is a reduction in accommodative function that develops with advancing age. Emmetropia is normal vision. (**Ref. 2,** p. 938; **Ref. 78,** p. 2211)

**411. (A)** Age-related macular degeneration is the leading cause of blindness in individuals over 50 years of age in the United States. (**Ref. 81,** p. 1994)

**412. (A); 413. (B); 414. (A); 415. (D)** The common pairs of psychiatric disorders occurring in the general population are alcoholism with drug abuse or antisocial behavior, obsessive-compulsive personality with panic disorder, and depression with somatization. (**Ref. 2,** p. 955)

**416.** **(D)** Forklift operators, fire fighters, and blast furnace workers are at risk for carbon monoxide poisoning. The symptoms of carbon monoxide toxicity include cognitive disturbances in concentration and memory, impulsivity, and lack of insight into one's behavior. (**Ref. 2,** p. 955)

**417.** **(B)** Health problems associated with high levels of family conflict, abuse, or neglect include depression, sleep disorders, phobias, generalized anxiety, antisocial behavior, school behavior problems, and developmental delay. (**Ref. 2,** p. 954)

**418.** **(D)** Women who lack a confiding relationship with their husbands, are not employed outside the home, have three or more children, or experienced the loss of their parents during childhood have a higher risk of depression. (**Ref. 2,** p. 953)

**419.** **(C)** Studies of patients with chronic diseases have identified persons with multiple sclerosis, cancer, diabetes mellitus, cardiovascular disease, thyroid disease, and chronic pain as reporting high rates of depression. (**Ref. 2,** p. 952)

**420.** **(B)** This patient most likely has post-traumatic stress disorder (PTSD). Persons with PTSD have symptoms such as sleep disturbance, survivor guilt, difficulty concentrating, hyperalertness, avoidance of activities associated with the event, and an intensification of symptoms if reexposed to a similar event. These patients also relive the traumatic event(s) through recurrent thoughts or dreams. (**Ref. 2,** p. 952)

**421.** **(B)** Prevention reduces the incidence of mental retardation, and medical care, being more effective than it was, increases its prevalence by helping people live longer. (**Ref. 2,** p. 963)

**422.** **(C)** In terms of mental retardation, impairment refers to an underlying biologic disorder; disability refers to a deficit in function; and handicap refers to social role and status. (**Ref. 2,** p. 963)

**423.** **(D)** On a normally distributed curve, 68% of the population is within 1 standard deviation of the mean; 95% are within 2 standard deviations; and 99.9% are within 3 standard deviations of the mean. Thus, for the given example, 2.5% of the population will score below 70. (**Ref. 2,** p. 966)

**424.** **(A)**  The Oregon group exemplifies in raw data form the prediction that 2.5% of the population will score below 70 based on a normally distributed curve with a mean of 100 and a standard deviation of 15. (**Ref. 2,** p. 966)

**425.** **(C)**  For autosomal recessive disorders, both parents are unaffected carriers. Of their children, 25% will be affected, 25% will not have the gene, and 50% will be unaffected carriers. (**Ref. 2,** pp. 966, 967)

**426.** **(C)**  Maternal exposure to alcohol during pregnancy results in fetal alcohol syndrome associated with mental retardation, low birth weight, narrow palpebral fissures, microcephaly, and flattened nasolabial facies. (**Ref. 2,** p. 968)

**427.** **(D)**  Syphilis, rubella, cytomegalovirus, and toxoplasmosis are all capable of causing congenital defects with prenatal infection. (**Ref. 2,** pp. 968, 969)

**428.** **(A)**  Ingestion of lead by a young child can lead to a severe encephalopathy and sometimes death. The most common source is lead from paint on toys or peeling from poorly maintained older housing. (**Ref. 2,** p. 969)

**429.** **(C)**  Sporadic cretinism as a result of congenital hypothyroidism is caused by severe iodine deficiency. (**Ref. 2,** p. 969)

**430.** **(C)**  Among community-based elderly, the most common ADL dependencies included bathing and transferring with assistance, with eating being least common. (**Ref. 2,** p. 973)

**431.** **(A)**  There is a strong association between ADL limitation and the presence of chronic medical conditions. Stroke and hip fracture have been shown to be directly related to specific disabilities. (**Ref. 2,** p. 973)

**432.** **(B)**  Based on the presumed thesis, future prevalence rates of disability and chronic care would be expected to diminish relative to current rates. (**Ref. 2,** p. 974)

**433.** **(A)** Based on this thesis, future prevalence rates of disability and chronic care would be expected to increase relative to current rates. **(Ref. 2, p. 974)**

**434.** **(D)** Age-related biologic changes in the elderly include a decrease in bone density, modification of lens protein leading to cataracts and loss of vision, stiffening of arterial walls, and a decrease in maximum oxygen consumption. **(Ref. 2, p. 975)**

**435.** **(C)** Osteoporosis is accentuated in postmenopausal women and is significantly reduced by estrogen replacement therapy. **(Ref. 2, p. 977)**

**436.** **(D)** The symptoms describe urge incontinence when urine is lost because of uninhibited bladder muscle contractions, usually resulting from a local bladder irritation or stroke. **(Ref. 2, p. 978)**

**437.** **(C)** Urinalysis. **(Ref. 2, p. 978)**

**438.** **(A)** If treatment of a urinary tract infection does not stop the incontinence, anticholinergic agents may be used. **(Ref. 2, p. 978)**

**439.** **(C)** The symptoms describe Parkinson's disease. **(Ref. 2, p. 979)**

**440.** **(D)** A deficiency in dopamine is associated with Parkinson's disease. **(Ref. 2, p. 979)**

**441.** **(B)** All neuroleptics should be discontinued. **(Ref. 2, p. 979)**

**442.** **(A)** Physical therapy should be instituted. **(Ref. 2, p. 979)**

**443.** **(D)** The 1989 RDAs recommend intake levels for protein, 11 vitamins, and 7 minerals according to age, body size, gender, and developmental stage. **(Ref. 2, p. 995)**

**444.** **(B)** RDAs are established at levels that exceed the nutritional requirements of 97% of the population; thus, they are designed to prevent deficiencies. **(Ref. 2, p. 995)**

**445.** **(A)** Pyridoxine deficiency is characterized by seborrheic skin lesions about the eyes, nose, and mouth. INH interferes with the uptake of pyridoxine. Pyridoxine deficiency is more prominent in patients who are alcoholics and are on INH. (**Ref. 80,** p. 1539)

**446.** (**D**) Malnutrition causes the loss of cellular immune competence. Malnourished children demonstrate poor resistance to infectious diseases. Infections, in turn, increase nutrient losses, leading to further malnutrition. This cycle is the principal cause of death among young children in developing countries. (**Ref. 2,** p. 996)

**447.** (**B**) "Baby-bottle" tooth decay is most prevalent in the maxillary incisors. It is characterized by rapid development of caries in the primary teeth caused by prolonged tooth contact with cariogenic substances such as milk sweetened with sugar, sugared water, fruit juices, or carbonated beverages taken from a bottle or pacifier. Native Americans have an extremely high prevalence of "baby-bottle" caries. (**Ref. 2,** pp. 1006, 1008)

**448.** (**D**) For children age 6 months to 3 years old, no fluoride supplementation is recommended if the child's water supply has at least 0.3 ppm fluoride concentration. For children age 3 to 6, the recommended supplementation is 0.25 mg per day, and for children 6 to 16, the amount is 0.50 mg per day. (**Ref. 76**)

**449.** (**D**) Methods of preventing periodontal disease include tooth brushing, flossing, and rinsing one's mouth with Listerine or Peridex. The value of these methods is in reducing plaque. (**Ref. 2,** p. 1015)

**450.** (**A**) The leading cause of potential years of life lost before age 65 in the United States is unintentional injury, followed by malignancy and intentional injury. (**Ref. 79**)

**451.** (**B**) Consumption of alcohol and drugs has been associated with all forms of homicide except child homicide. (**Ref. 2,** p. 1037)

**452.** (**A**) Central injuries, blows to the chest and abdomen, should raise the suspicion of battering. Battering can prompt a range of medical and psychosocial problems such as rape, attempted suicide, and psychotic breaks. (**Ref. 2,** p. 1042)

**453. (D)** Many children who witness violence suffer from post-traumatic stress disorder. Children who suffer abuse show delays in physical, social, and emotional development. **(Ref. 2, p.** 1038)

**454. (B)** Drug overdose is the most common form of suicide for females aged 15 to 24. For males the method is shooting, followed by hanging. **(Ref. 2, p.** 1054)

**455. (A)** The long-term psychologic effects of child abuse include a propensity to aggression in adolescence, language disorders, and lower performance on standardized tests of intelligence. **(Ref. 2, p.** 1047)

**456. (D)** Former cigarette smokers experience declining mortality rates as the years of not smoking increase. Overall mortality rates for female smokers are less than for male smokers. However, tests of women with smoking characteristics similar to those of men indicate mortality rates similar to those of male smokers. Mortality rates are decreased in smokers who use cigarettes with decreased tar and nicotine content. **(Ref. 84, pp.** 38–41, 43–46)

**457. (B)** Lung cancer mortality rates are increasing more rapidly in women than in men, and this is why lung cancer has now surpassed cancer of the breast as the leading cause of cancer deaths in women. **(Ref. 84, p.** 21)

**458. (B)** Low back pain is the most expensive occupational health problem in the United States. **(Ref. 85, p.** 342)

**459. (D)** Falls account for almost half of the accidental deaths in the home. Fire burns rank second. **(Ref. 86, p.** 1558)

**460. (B)** Average annual age-specific unintentional injury peaks at ages 15 through 25. Males have higher death rates than females at all ages. Blacks and Native Americans have higher rates than whites and Asians in all major categories except falls. **(Ref. 2, pp.** 1023, 1024)

**461. (A)** Motor vehicle accidents account for greater than half of unintentional injury deaths in the United States. **(Ref. 2, p.** 1024)

**462. (B)** The most frequent cause of house fires is a cigarette dropped on bedding or upholstered furniture. Lower ignitions by cigarettes are associated with low tobacco density, low circumference, lower paper porosity, and no citrate added. Application of all possible modifications would achieve up to 75% reduction in cigarette-related injuries. **(Ref. 2, p. 1031)**

**463. (B)** In comparison with Sweden and the Netherlands, the US infant mortality rates are much higher. In 1975 the US rate was 16.1 per 1000 live births, Sweden 8.3, and the Netherlands 10.6, respectively. The difference in IMR between races is related to a large extent to the differences in incidence of low birth weight. **(Ref. 87, pp. 1704–1705)**

**464. (C)** In 1987 accidents ranked fourth as a cause of overall death, a position that has been maintained for many years. **(Ref. 86, p. 9)**

**465. (B)** Accidents are the leading cause of death among all persons aged 1 to 38; for youths 15 to 24 years old, accidents claim about four times more lives than the next leading cause. **(Ref. 86, p. 8)**

**466. (D)** Calculations by the Centers for Disease Control focusing upon years of potential life lost (YPLL) before age 65 goes beyond absolute causes of death to those that deprive people of the best years of their lives. "Unintentional injuries" includes accidents and adverse effects. **(Ref. 87, p. 20)**

**467. (B)** Accidental death rates from 1976–1986 dropped for every age category, down 16%. The smallest drop was 10% for 25 to 44 years of age; the greatest was 34% for under 5 years. **(Ref. 86, p. 16–18)**

**468. (A)** On November 4, 1986, Massachusetts became the first state to repeal its mandatory seat belt use law. A survey of voters found that the most common reason for voting against the law was that it was an infringement on personal freedom; belief that the law was ineffective was the second most common reason given. **(Ref. 88, pp. 548–552)**

**469. (C)** In Nebraska, child restraint device usage dropped from 62% to 42% following repeal of the law requiring adults to use seat belts, despite the fact that the state still required child restraint use. (**Ref. 86,** p. 53)

**470. (D)** In 1986 alcohol was a factor in at least 21,000 motor vehicle accident fatalities, about 320,000 injury accidents, and about 1,300,000 property damage accidents. The estimated annual cost of alcohol-related motor vehicle accidents is about $12 billion. (**Ref. 86,** p. 52)

**471. (B)** NHSTA defines a BAC of greater than 0.01 g/dL but less than 0.10 g/dL as indicating a low level of alcohol and a BAC of greater than 0.10 g/dL (the legal level of intoxication in most states) as indicating intoxication. (**Ref. 16,** p. 889)

**472. (C)** Motorcycles, motor scooters, and motorbikes constituted 3% of 1986 vehicle registrations but were involved in 8% of the fatal accidents. Trucks constituted 22% of registrations and were involved in 26% of fatal accidents. (**Ref. 86,** p. 60)

**473. (D)** The injury total of 3,100,000 means that one person in 78 was disabled 1 or more days by injuries received in home accidents in 1986. About 80,000 of these injuries resulted in some permanent impairment. (**Ref. 86,** p. 87)

**474. (A)** The death rate for agricultural workers was 52/100,000 in 1986 compared to 50/100,000 for mining and quarrying, 33/100,000 for construction, 27/100,000 for transportation and public utilities, and 6/100,000 for manufacturing. (**Ref. 86,** p. 29)

**475. (E)** By the age of 65, the probability of lung cancer decreases, but prostate cancer continues to increase, affecting older men and especially blacks. The reader should be cautious to discern between cancer morbidity and cancer mortality when interpreting these statements. (**Ref. 88,** pp. 11–15)

# 4

# Environmental Health Issues

**DIRECTIONS:** Each of the numbered items or incomplete statements in this section is followed by answers or completions of the statement. Select the **ONE** lettered answer or completion that is **BEST** in each case.

**476.** Following cigarette smoking, what is the second leading cause of lung cancer in the United States?
   **A.** Coal mining
   **B.** Exposure to asbestos
   **C.** Exposure to radon
   **D.** Air pollution
   **E.** Environmental or secondhand tobacco smoke exposure

**477.** Neurologic effects can follow ingestion of various toxic substances. Symptoms of tremors, emotional lability, neurasthesis, and psychomotor disturbances can be caused by which of the following toxic substances?
   **A.** Lead
   **B.** Arsenic
   **C.** Mercury
   **D.** Aromatic solvents
   **E.** Malathion

**Questions 478 and 479:**
A 60-year-old white woman presents with shortness of breath on exertion that has been present for 3 months, and has been gradually worsening. She is a nonsmoker. Her husband died 10 years previously from lung cancer. He had smoked one pack of cigarettes per day for over 30 years. He worked for over 30 years as an insulator. On lung examination, decreased breath sounds are heard throughout her lung fields. Wheezing is present on forced expiration.

**478.** A chest roentgenogram is ordered. What would be the most likely findings, based on the history and examination?
    **A.** Granulomatous changes in the upper lung fields
    **B.** Irregular opacities in the lower lung fields
    **C.** Bilateral loculated pleural effusions
    **D.** Lobar infiltrates in the lower lung fields
    **E.** Hilar enlargement

**479.** What would be the most likely cause of mortality for this woman, related to the history and examination findings?
    **A.** Mesothelioma
    **B.** Asbestosis
    **C.** Lung cancer
    **D.** Bacterial pneumonia
    **E.** Chronic obstructive pulmonary disease

**480.** Exposure to asbestos can result in pulmonary fibrosis. What is the mechanism by which this occurs?
    **A.** Macrophages phagocytize asbestos fibrils and then release factors such as fibronectin
    **B.** Asbestos fibrils migrate to the pleural space, causing fibrosis while working through tissue
    **C.** Asbestos fibrils migrate into the lymphatic system and cause obstruction
    **D.** Asbestos fibers become coated with hemosiderin and form asbestos bodies
    **E.** Asbestos fibers form the nidus for infection

**Questions 481 and 482:**
Match the pulmonary disorders with the changes in pulmonary function tests usually found for that disorder.

| Forced expiratory volume in 1 second ($FEV_1$) | Total lung capacity (TLC) |
|---|---|
| **A.** decreased | normal or increased |
| **B.** decreased | decreased |

**481.** Asbestosis

**482.** Complicated coal worker's pneumoconiosis

**Questions 483 and 484:**
A 45-year-old man who has been a coal worker for 20 years presents with dyspnea that started 6 months ago and has grown progressively worse. He is a nonsmoker. He has had a chronic cough for nearly 12 months. He is a poor historian and unaware of what previous examinations have shown. He states that he had always felt fine up until about 1 year ago. Examination of the lungs shows mild wheezing on forced expiration, with a slightly increased expiratory phase.

**483.** A chest roentgenogram is performed. What findings are likely, on the basis of the history and examination?
A. Lobar infiltrates in the lower lung fields
B. Pleural thickening laterally
C. Hilar and mediastinal adenopathy
D. Multiple small rounded opacities
E. Granulomatous disease

**484.** For what additional pulmonary pathology is this man at increased risk?
A. Pleural effusion
B. Mesothelioma
C. Adenocarcinoma of the lung
D. *Mycobacterium tuberculosis* infection
E. Pneumonia

**485.** With what cancer is coal worker's pneumoconiosis associated?
  **A.** Lung cancer
  **B.** Gastric cancer
  **C.** Colon cancer
  **D.** Bladder cancer
  **E.** Kidney cancer

**486.** A long-time employee for the steel industry has developed deep, painless ulcers of the knuckles and nail roots, contact dermatitis of the hands, and corrosion of the nasal mucous membranes. Exposure to which of the following is most likely?
  **A.** Magnesium
  **B.** Chromium
  **C.** Cobalt
  **D.** Copper
  **E.** Nickel

**Questions 487–491:**
Match the chemicals with the following descriptions.

  **A.** mercury
  **B.** chromium
  **C.** lead
  **D.** iron

**487.** A well-documented carcinogen and one of the best-known allergens in the occupational environment.

**488.** Associated with the most prevalent metal deficiency syndrome in humans.

**489.** Chronic overload leads to hemosiderosis and liver cirrhosis.

**490.** Chronic effects on red blood cells and the nervous system are clinically important in toxicity of this metal.

**491.** Acute poisoning causes chemical pneumonitis and pulmonary edema.

**492.** Radon exposure in uranium miners is known to cause which of the following?
   **A.** Chemical pneumonitis
   **B.** Lung cancer
   **C.** Violent sneezing, dyspnea, and wheezing
   **D.** Hodgkin's disease
   **E.** Lymphoma

**493.** Earlobe dermatitis and hand eczema in a teenage girl is likely to be an allergy to
   **A.** copper
   **B.** nickel
   **C.** brass
   **D.** silver
   **E.** magnesium

**494.** A 56-year-old black man, employed at a battery repair shop, is brought to the hospital by his wife because of his failing health. After a history, clinical examination, and laboratory tests, which of the following are likely to be found?
   **A.** Poor concentration, memory, and attention span
   **B.** Elevated hemoglobin and low serum bilirubin
   **C.** Pulmonary infiltrates on chest roentgenogram
   **D.** Positive hemocult test
   **E.** 15 to 20 RBCs/HPF on urinalysis

**495.** A 28-year-old white man, employed as a sandblaster, has a 3-day history of abdominal pain, weakness, fatigue, pallor and a hemoglobin of 7.6 g/dL, low mean corpuscular volume (MCV), and low mean corpuscular hemoglobin concentration (MCHC). The most likely diagnosis is
   **A.** magnesium deficiency
   **B.** selenium deficiency
   **C.** excessive intake of cobalt
   **D.** classic lead poisoning
   **E.** Wilson's disease

**Questions 496–501:**
Certain human diseases have been traced to exposure to environmental and occupational chemicals. Match the following. Each may be used once, more than once, or not at all.

A. asbestos
B. mercury
C. silicon dioxide
D. benzene
E. carbon tetrachloride

**496.** 4-cm coin lesion in the left midlung field on chest roentgenogram (CXR)

**497.** Elevated lactic dehydrogenase (LDH), asparate aminotransferase (AST), and alanine amino transferase (ALT)

**498.** Pleural effusion and pleural plaque on CXR

**499.** White blood cell (WBC) count of 86,000

**500.** Tremors of the upper extremities, irritability, and difficulty concentrating

**501.** Several discrete round opacities 1 to 3 mm in diameter in upper lung fields on CXR

**502.** Common sources of lead in the environment include all of the following **EXCEPT**
A. pasteurized milk
B. drinking water
C. canned foods
D. garden vegetables
E. emissions from metal smelters

**503.** The primary source of radon exposure in the home is
A. off-gassing from formaldehyde in carpets and furniture
B. from underground through cracks and seams in building structures
C. breakdown of insecticides applied to moist areas under sinks
D. emissions from closets containing freshly dry-cleaned garments
E. gas stoves

**504.** It is estimated that 50 deaths occur annually in the United States from accidental ingestion of
   A. isopropyl alcohol
   B. ethylene glycol
   C. fluorocarbons
   D. methyl chloroform
   E. methyl bromide

**505.** If an oral thermometer were to break in the mouth, swallowing the inorganic mercury would cause
   A. hypochromic microcytic anemia
   B. no health effects
   C. central and peripheral neuropathy
   D. deafness and vision problems
   E. acute renal failure

**506.** Health effects of lead include
   A. disrupts heme synthesis
   B. gastrointestinal pain
   C. direct axonal damage
   D. encephalopathy with seizures
   E. all of the above

**507.** The following are true of organophosphate pesticides **EXCEPT**
   A. cause inhibition of acetylcholinesterase
   B. poisoning can be treated with atropine
   C. parathion is responsible for most of the occupational poisonings and deaths in the United States
   D. pralidoxime (2-PAM) can reactivate cholinesterase if given within 7 days of poisoning
   E. parathion is the most common pesticide cause of death

**508.** Chlorinated hydrocarbons
   A. are peripheral nervous system stimulants
   B. are lipophobic
   C. cause generalized seizures
   D. biodegrade quickly
   E. are food additives

**509.** The usual cause of death with paraquat is
   **A.** pulmonary fibrosis
   **B.** myocardial failure
   **C.** hepatic failure
   **D.** renal failure
   **E.** status epilepticus

**510.** The usual cause of death from fumigants is
   **A.** hepatotoxicity
   **B.** neurotoxicity
   **C.** toxic psychosis
   **D.** pulmonary edema
   **E.** congestive heart failure

**511.** Persons exposed to pesticides show increased risk for all of the following **EXCEPT**
   **A.** brain cancer
   **B.** leukemia
   **C.** colon cancer
   **D.** lung cancer
   **E.** non-Hodgkin's lymphoma

**512.** Major factors affecting thermoregulation include all of the following **EXCEPT**
   **A.** heat production by metabolism
   **B.** heat loss by evaporation
   **C.** heat loss or gain via convection
   **D.** heat loss through stress
   **E.** heat loss or gain via radiation

**513.** Heat stroke is characterized by
   **A.** clear mental status
   **B.** sweating possibly absent or diminished
   **C.** elevation of core body temperature usually no more than 102°F
   **D.** treatment directed at slow lowering of temperature
   **E.** normal body temperature

**514.** Heat exhaustion is characterized by
    **A.** body temperature rarely normal
    **B.** development within hours, as a rule
    **C.** dizziness and weakness
    **D.** primarily gastrointestinal symptoms, ie, nausea and vomiting
    **E.** seizure disorder

**515.** Heat syncope is characterized by
    **A.** a transient fall in blood pressure with an associated loss of consciousness
    **B.** muscle cramps
    **C.** nausea
    **D.** shortness of breath
    **E.** pulmonary edema

**516.** The following is true about heat-related deaths.
    **A.** Excess mortality occurs in suburban areas
    **B.** Infants and children are at less risk
    **C.** Obese are at increased risk
    **D.** Death rates are higher in women when compared with men
    **E.** The elderly are at less risk

**517.** Important components of occupational surveillance for disease and injury are
    **A.** detection and enumeration of morbidity and mortality
    **B.** data evaluation and interpretation
    **C.** intervention
    **D.** only A and B
    **E.** A, B, and C

**518.** Specific activities conducted on an occupational health surveillance program include all of the following **EXCEPT**
    **A.** medical screening
    **B.** medical monitoring
    **C.** biological monitoring
    **D.** exposure monitoring
    **E.** work productivity

**519.** The leading work-related disease category is
    **A.** occupational lung disease
    **B.** musculoskeletal injuries

**C.** occupational cancer
**D.** cardiovascular disease
**E.** infectious diseases

**520.** Among the most common causes of work-related diseases are all of the following **EXCEPT**
   **A.** traumatic injuries
   **B.** reproductive disorders
   **C.** noise induced hearing loss
   **D.** skin diseases
   **E.** endocrinological disorders

**521.** Neurotoxic disorders include
   **A.** peripheral neuropathy
   **B.** personality changes
   **C.** toxic encephalitis
   **D.** sciatica
   **E.** psychoses

**522.** Testing to diagnose disease in individuals at an early stage is
   **A.** medical screening
   **B.** medical monitoring
   **C.** biologic monitoring
   **D.** exposure monitoring
   **E.** disease monitoring

**523.** Name the act that prohibits employment discrimination against a qualified individual because of a disability.
   **A.** Equal Employment Opportunity
   **B.** Right to Privacy
   **C.** Rehabilitation Act
   **D.** Civil Rights Act
   **E.** Affirmative Action

**524.** Percentage of adults who are work-disabled is
   **A.** 20%
   **B.** 15%
   **C.** 11%
   **D.** 5%
   **E.** 1%

**525.** Select the race with the highest prevalence of disabilities.
  **A.** White
  **B.** African-American
  **C.** Native American
  **D.** Asian-American
  **E.** Iranian-American

**526.** The age group with the most likelihood of disabilities is
  **A.** 16 to 20-year-olds
  **B.** 25 to 34-year-olds
  **C.** 35 to 44-year-olds
  **D.** 45 to 54-year-olds
  **E.** 55 to 64-year-olds

**Questions 527 and 528:**
Match the following.

  **A.** inverse relationship to disabilities
  **B.** proportional relationship to disabilities
  **C.** slight relationship to disabilities
  **D.** insignificant relationship to disabilities
  **E.** no relationship to disabilities

**527.** Income has a/an

**528.** Educational level has a/an

**529.** The first step in conducting a rational assessment of one's ability to do a job is
  **A.** job analysis
  **B.** job surveillance
  **C.** physical exam
  **D.** exercise treadmill test
  **E.** trial at position

**530.** Acute health effects of pesticide exposure include all of the following **EXCEPT**
  **A.** diarrhea
  **B.** dehydration
  **C.** weakness
  **D.** headaches
  **E.** listlessness

**531.** Indicate the state that mandates physician reporting of pesticide-related illness.
  **A.** New York
  **B.** Oklahoma
  **C.** Iowa
  **D.** California
  **E.** Illinois

**532.** The most common work-related health care problem in agriculture is
  **A.** dermatitis
  **B.** gastroenteritis
  **C.** eczema
  **D.** seizure disorder
  **E.** renal failure

**533.** Inadequate sanitation for farm workers leads to all of the following **EXCEPT**
  **A.** heat stress
  **B.** pesticide-related illness
  **C.** constipation
  **D.** urinary tract infections
  **E.** communicable diseases

**534.** An increased incidence of cancer in the African-American population is thought to be due to
  **A.** lifestyle factors
  **B.** employment in American industry, with resultant increase in occupational cancer
  **C.** environmental exposures
  **D.** genetic variables
  **E.** ingestion of Nutrasweet

**535.** Noise causes the following **EXCEPT**
  **A.** hearing loss
  **B.** adverse affects on children's language development
  **C.** clinical depression
  **D.** alterations in immune system
  **E.** hindrance of performance of tasks requiring high levels of accuracy

**536.** Noise-induced hearing loss is often preceded by
   A. tinnitus
   B. intermittent hearing loss
   C. Meniere's disease
   D. upper respiratory infection
   E. coughing

**537.** Prevention of noise-induced hearing loss includes all of the following **EXCEPT**
   A. reduction of the noise in the workplace
   B. noise restriction on equipment implemented
   C. ear defenders
   D. job rotation
   E. screening for low-frequency loss

**538.** Frequency range that is essential for perception of speech is
   A. 300 to 4000 Hz
   B. 100 to 250 Hz
   C. 400 to 5000 Hz
   D. 5000 to 7000 Hz
   E. 7500 to 9000 Hz

**539.** Sociocucus is hearing loss resulting from
   A. loud noises
   B. old age
   C. a genetic disorder
   D. otitis media
   E. sinusitis

**540.** Presbycusis is hearing loss resulting from
   A. a bacterial ear infection
   B. loud noises
   C. old age
   D. blockage via excess earwax
   E. prematurity

**541.** Temporary threshold shift
   A. is age-dependent
   B. never becomes permanent hearing loss
   C. usually lasts a few days
   D. occurs after a loud noise
   E. is usually one-sided

**542.** Occupational Safety and Health Administration (OSHA) does all the following **EXCEPT**
A. makes safety and health standards
B. conducts inspections and investigations
C. issues citations and imposes penalties
D. does not require employers to keep a record of safety
E. petition courts to restrain imminent danger situations

**543.** The National Institute for Occupational Safety and Health (NIOSH)
A. monitors compliance with employment laws
B. educates professionals through grants programs
C. does work-site investigations at the request of employers
D. establishes work-site standards
E. promotes occupational safety legislation

**Questions 544–547:**
Match each of the following organizations with their responsibilities.

A. Occupational Safety and Health Administration (OSHA)
B. United States Department of Agriculture (USDA)
C. Food and Drug Administration (FDA)
D. World Health Organization (WHO) and Food and Agriculture Organization (FAO)

**544.** international food standards

**545.** food safety in the United States

**546.** protection for agricultural workers

**547.** inspection, grading, and certification of agricultural products

**548.** The following etiologic agents are responsible for the majority of outbreaks of food-borne illness.
A. Viruses
B. Bacteria
C. Chemicals
D. Parasites
E. None of the above

**549.** Heat stable enterotoxin is produced by which one of the following?
A. *Staphylococcus aureus*
B. *Campylobacter* species
C. *Listeria monocytogenes*
D. *Salmonella* species
E. *Vibrio parahaemolyticus*

**550.** Which of the following is most commonly associated with botulism in the United States?
A. Fish
B. Pork
C. Rice
D. Home-canned vegetables and fruit
E. Seafood

**551.** The etiologic agent most often responsible for food-borne disease in the United States is
A. *Clostridium perfringens*
B. *Salmonella* species
C. *Staphylococcus aureus*
D. *Campylobacter jejuni*
E. *Yersinia enterocolitica*

**552.** Sanitary control of food production may involve all of the following **EXCEPT**
A. proper temperature and relative humidity
B. irradiation
C. ethylene bromide
D. design of storage facility
E. protection from moisture

**553.** Illnesses related to dairy products have been associated with all of the following agents **EXCEPT**
A. *Listeria monocytogenes*
B. *Campylobacter jejuni*
C. *Yersinia enterocolitica*
D. *Bacillus cereus*
E. *Staphylococcus aureus*

**554.** The methods of sanitizing food-processing equipment include all the following **EXCEPT**
A. chlorine
B. radiation
C. potassium permanganate
D. heat
E. iodine compounds

**555.** Which of the following is the most effective method for inhibiting bacterial growth?
A. Dehydration
B. Freezing to less than 10°C
C. Refrigeration at 4 to 7°C
D. Blanching
E. Dairy fermentations

**556.** Studies have shown that the most important contributing factor for confirmed food-borne disease outbreaks is
A. unsafe time–temperature relationships
B. food from an unsafe source
C. contaminated equipment
D. poor personal hygiene
E. inadequate cooking

**557.** What is the most common vehicle for transmission of *Staphylococcus aureus*?
A. Cream-filled pastries
B. Pork
C. Chicken and mixed salads
D. Turkey
E. Beef

**Questions 558–561:**
Match the following options with the associated activity. Each option can be used once, more than once, or not at all.

    **A.** Delaney clause
    **B.** Generally Recognized As Safe (GRAS) list
    **C.** Codex Alimentarius Commission
    **D.** Pasteurized Milk Ordinance (PMO)

**558.** Inspection of production, transportation, and processing facilities and testing of raw and pasteurized milk

**559.** Guidelines on international food standards

**560.** Food substance that has been found to cause cancer in humans or animals

**561.** Incidental and intentional food additives excluding substances found to be of questionable safety

**562.** The single largest use of residential water is in
    **A.** laundry
    **B.** toilet flushing
    **C.** bathing
    **D.** drinking and cooking
    **E.** dishwashing

**563.** The following features are related to groundwater **EXCEPT**
    **A.** highly mineralized
    **B.** higher sanitary quality than surface water
    **C.** recharges by rainwater and runoff through the ground
    **D.** has opportunity for coagulation and sedimentation
    **E.** improved bacteriologic quality as compared to surface water

**564.** What is the primary source of fresh water?
    **A.** Groundwater
    **B.** Lake water
    **C.** Rainwater
    **D.** Surface water
    **E.** Ocean water

**565.** What percent of the water in the world is fresh water readily available for use?
- **A.** 10%
- **B.** 1%
- **C.** 0.2%
- **D.** 0.8%
- **E.** 0.06%

**566.** The most important contributor to surface water degradation is
- **A.** exposure to sunlight
- **B.** coagulation and sedimentation of colloidal and suspended solid particles
- **C.** eutrophication
- **D.** attenuation of high levels of contaminants
- **E.** addition of rainwater

**567.** Asbestos exposure has been associated with all of the following **EXCEPT**
- **A.** peritoneal mesothelioma
- **B.** gastrointestinal tract cancers
- **C.** lung cancer
- **D.** breast cancer
- **E.** pleural mesothelioma

**568.** What percent of groundwater supplies have detectable radon?
- **A.** 85%
- **B.** 70%
- **C.** 50%
- **D.** 25%
- **E.** 20%

**569.** The following water-borne diseases are commonly associated with ingestion of water **EXCEPT**
- **A.** cryptosporidiosis
- **B.** schistosomiasis
- **C.** adenoviruses
- **D.** hepatitis A
- **E.** polio

**570.** Which of the following has been the most important process for assuring bacteriologic safety of potable water?
  **A.** Filtration
  **B.** Chlorine
  **C.** Iodine
  **D.** Sedimentation
  **E.** Coagulation

**571.** The following are all methods of commercial water disinfection **EXCEPT**
  **A.** ferric salts
  **B.** mercury vapor arc lamp
  **C.** silver ions
  **D.** copper ions
  **E.** irradiation by ultraviolet light

**572.** The best measure that evaluates whether a body of water remains aerobic or anaerobic in relation to organic wastes typical of human discharges is
  **A.** coliform count
  **B.** carbon dioxide levels
  **C.** biochemical oxygen demand
  **D.** total organic carbon
  **E.** bacterial cultures

**Questions 573–576:**
Match each of the following results with the water source or content. Each of the options can be used once, more than once, or not at all.

  **A.** methemoglobinemia
  **B.** cardiovascular disease mortality
  **C.** laxative effect
  **D.** affects sodium concentration of water

**573.** Sulfates in drinking water

**574.** Well water

**575.** Hard water

**576.** Softening of water by ion exchange

**577.** The minimum safe distance of a latrine or privy from a well can be predicted with each of the following **EXCEPT**
   A. direction of groundwater flow
   B. nature of the soil
   C. limestone content of soil
   D. distance from groundwater
   E. height of groundwater

**578.** Chlorination of effluents in waste-water treatment may do all of the following **EXCEPT**
   A. be toxic to aquatic life
   B. cause proliferation of beneficial microorganisms
   C. produce chlorinated hydrocarbons
   D. be required where effluents are discharged to water used for shellfish growing
   E. destroy pathogens

**579.** Waste-water reclamation has been used for all of the following **EXCEPT**
   A. irrigation in agriculture
   B. cooling in industry
   C. residential consumption
   D. recreational lakes
   E. urban irrigation

**580.** The dominant method of solid waste disposal in the United States is
   A. incineration
   B. landfill
   C. recycling
   D. composting
   E. dumping at sea

**581.** Incineration is associated with all of the following **EXCEPT**
   A. stabilizing hazardous material
   B. causing ground subsidence over time
   C. turning perishable organic material to inorganic material
   D. reducing waste quantity by up to one fifteenth to one twentieth
   E. killing pathogenic organisms

**582.** The main problem gas in municipal solid waste incineration is
- **A.** sulfuric acid
- **B.** hydrogen chloride
- **C.** hydrogen fluoride
- **D.** mercury
- **E.** nitrogen oxide

**Questions 583–586:**
Match each of the following recycling options with the most appropriate material. Each of the options may be used once, more than once, or not at all.

- **A.** recovery and transformation into raw material for remanufacture
- **B.** recycling with energy recovery
- **C.** recovery and reuse as new
- **D.** recovery with conversion of the recovered material

**583.** Kitchen garbage

**584.** Combustible and nonhazardous waste

**585.** Glass bottles

**586.** Aluminum cans

**587.** The most important exposure pathway from radioactive disposal facilities is
- **A.** surface water
- **B.** ingestion of drinking water
- **C.** groundwater
- **D.** swimming in lake water
- **E.** stream water

**588.** Ozone attains maximum density at an altitude of approximately
- **A.** 5 km
- **B.** 22 km
- **C.** 36 km
- **D.** 53 km
- **E.** 75 km

**589.** As one ascends in altitude, the density of the air does which one of the following?
A. Increases linearly
B. Decreases linearly
C. Increases exponentially
D. Decreases exponentially
E. Does not change

**590.** A pilot flying at an altitutde of 2500 meters experiences drowsiness, finds calculations difficult, and has difficulty with seeing in the dark. What is the reason for his symptoms?
A. Alcohol intoxication
B. Hypoglycemia
C. Vitamin A deficiency
D. Hyperglycemia
E. Hypoxia

**591.** Which of the following is the most important modality for providing us input to maintain spatial orientation?
A. Vestibular function
B. Vision
C. Proprioception
D. Motion
E. Tactile sense

**592.** Each of the following are factors of concern in *both* high altitude flying and the space environment **EXCEPT**
A. reduced availability of oxygen
B. reduced atmospheric pressure
C. ionizing radiation
D. thermal extremes
E. changes in gravity

**593.** In space flights, biomedical effects include all of the following **EXCEPT**
A. loss of red cell mass
B. decrease in bone mineral density
C. absence of motion sickness as a result of null gravity
D. cardiovascular system deconditioning
E. social deprivation

**594.** Which of the following levels of blood alcohol represent the lowest level found to adversely compromise flight performance of pilots?
- **A.** 0.008%
- **B.** 0.02%
- **C.** 0.04%
- **D.** 0.06%
- **E.** 0.08%

**595.** Which of the following is the most prevalent indoor environment in the world?
- **A.** High-rise apartment homes in urban areas
- **B.** Shanty settlements in urban areas
- **C.** Traditional huts in rural communities
- **D.** Industrial premises
- **E.** Residential homes in urban areas

**596.** Which one of the following sources of indoor pollution is a primary concern in developing countries?
- **A.** Asbestos fibers
- **B.** Tobacco smoke
- **C.** Burning fuel for cooking
- **D.** Building materials
- **E.** Carpet adhesive

**597.** Potential risk of cancer based on animal models has led to restricted building use of materials produced from which one of the following?
- **A.** Sulfur dioxide
- **B.** Nitrogen dioxide
- **C.** Benzene
- **D.** Ozone
- **E.** Formaldehyde

**Questions 598–601:**
Match each one of the following household settings with the most common mental health problem associated with it. Each option can be used once, more than once, or not at all.

- **A.** dormitory suburbs
- **B.** slums
- **C.** single-room rented apartments

**598.** Schizophrenia

**599.** Depression

**600.** Alcoholism

**601.** Adolescent delinquency and vandalism

**602.** Carbon dioxide, oxides of nitrogen, methane, chlorofluorocarbons, and ozone produced by human activities are associated with which one of the following?
A. Acid precipitation
B. Ozone depletion
C. Greenhouse effect
D. Indoor air pollution
E. Sludge digestion

**603.** At high latitudes, global warming could produce large amounts of methane as a result of which one of the following?
A. Agriculture work
B. Thawing permafrost
C. Coastal flooding
D. Annual monsoons
E. Industry

**604.** Probably the most important effect of ozone depletion is its direct adverse effect on which one of the following?
A. Humans
B. Rain forests
C. Agriculture
D. Plankton
E. Sea water

**605.** The principal pathologic lesions caused by the presence of asbestos in the lungs involve
A. the walls of terminal alveoli
B. membranous and respiratory bronchioles
C. ventral parietal pleura
D. perivenous lymphatic vessels
E. large airways

**606.** The anatomic measure of the severity of asbestosis is
 A. obstructive lesions of the small airways
 B. severely diminished vital capacity
 C. profusion of irregular opacities on chest roentgenogram
 D. a "small tight lung"
 E. asbestotic pleural plaques

**607.** The major public health concern and principal cause of death from asbestosis in developed countries is
 A. lung cancer
 B. rapidly spreading mesotheliomas that engulf vital organs
 C. pleural effusions and their sequelae
 D. severe airway obstruction
 E. neoplasms of the pharynx, larynx, and esophagus

**608.** The most effective method for prevention of coal worker's pneumoconiosis (CWP) is
 A. proper use of masks with coal-dust filters
 B. control of respirable coal-mine dust through proper ventilation of mining operations
 C. removal of miners with early evidence of CWP to low-dust jobs
 D. cessation of smoking among miners
 E. control of dust with special drilling procedures

**609.** Pathognomic signs or symptoms of CWP include
 A. chronic cough or phlegm in association with prolonged inhalation of coal dust
 B. progressive massive fibrosis
 C. characteristic radiographic opacities on chest film
 D. decreased $PaO_2$ together with obstructive and restrictive mechanical changes in the lung
 E. none of the above

**610.** CWP occurs in two forms, simple CWP and which of the following?
 A. Caplan's syndrome
 B. Combined silicosis and CWP
 C. Progressive massive fibrosis (PMF)
 D. Macronodular CWP
 E. CWP with hilar lymphadenopathy

**611.** The US Safe Drinking Water Act was enacted in 1974 to ensure safe drinking water supplies, protect purity of aquifers, and prevent groundwater contamination. In addition, the act requires the Environmental Protection Agency (EPA) to
  **A.** identify substances that contaminate drinking water and to set maximum contaminant levels (MCLs) for those substances
  **B.** ensure that states provide "fishable swimmable" waters
  **C.** regulate the bottled water trade
  **D.** monitor acid rain
  **E.** establish community water supplies

**612.** The Occupational Safety and Health Administration (OSHA) Hazard Communication Standard requires employers to inform workers of hazardous materials in the workplace. The scope of the standard requires the employer to do each of the following **EXCEPT**
  **A.** maintain materials safety data sheets
  **B.** ensure proper container labeling
  **C.** provide proper training on each hazardous chemical
  **D.** provide health care for affected workers
  **E.** maintain on-site medical evaluation capability

**613.** The Clean Air Act requires states to meet Primary and Secondary air quality standards. The Primary standards are set to protect general public health, whereas the Secondary standards are meant to
  **A.** protect individuals' preexisting health concerns
  **B.** protect infants and the elderly only
  **C.** protect livestock, crops, and structures
  **D.** avoid acid rain
  **E.** limit ozone depletion

**614.** The organization responsible for workplace health and safety enforcement activities is
  **A.** the National Institute for Occupational Safety and Health (NIOSH)
  **B.** the Occupational Safety and Health Administration (OSHA)
  **C.** the Occupational Safety and Health Review Commission (OSHRC)
  **D.** the American Industrial Hygiene Association (AIHA)
  **E.** the American Conference of Governmental Industrial Hygienists (ACGIH)

**615.** The Toxic Substance Control Act (TSCA)
   A. requires chemical manufacturers to conduct health-related tests on potentially hazardous substances
   B. empowers the EPA to remove substances from the marketplace that may cause unreasonable risk to human health or the environment
   C. regulates production, use, and disposal of hazardous products
   D. requires manufacturers to report results of testing and monitoring to the EPA
   E. all of the above

**616.** A worker exposed to methylene chloride during a paint-stripping operation would likely show evidence of which of the following?
   A. Elevated carboxyhemoglobin concentrations
   B. Elevated protoporphyrin in urine
   C. Plasma cholinesterase inhibition
   D. Low molecular weight proteinuria
   E. Elevated blood-zinc-protoporphyrin concentrations

**617.** Chemical exposures in the workplace may present a hazard to women and the infants they breast-feed. Toxic substances are passively transferred from plasma to breast milk if they
   A. are lipid soluble
   B. are polarized at body pH
   C. have low molecular weight
   D. all of the above
   E. none of the above are critical factors

**618.** Evidence suggests the most frequent US work-related infectious disease is
   A. histoplasmosis
   B. Newcastle disease
   C. hepatitis B
   D. rabies
   E. tuberculosis

**619.** Noise-induced hearing loss can usually be detected through audiometric examinations. Early impairment is usually detected at which frequency?
- **A.** 20 Hz
- **B.** 16,000 Hz
- **C.** 4000 Hz
- **D.** 12,000 Hz
- **E.** 8000- to 10,000-Hz range

**620.** Conductive hearing losses
- **A.** occur in the inner ear and are generally not correctable
- **B.** are caused by any condition that interferes with the transmission of sound through the external and middle ear and are generally not correctable
- **C.** are caused by any condition that interferes with the transmission of sound through the external and middle ear and are generally correctable
- **D.** are permanent losses resulting from damage of the auditory nerve
- **E.** occur as a result of cochlear hair cell damage

**621.** Chronic exposure to loud noise usually results in damage to the
- **A.** stapes
- **B.** inner ear, especially the organ of Corti
- **C.** oval window
- **D.** tympanic membrane
- **E.** pinna and external auditory canal

**622.** All of the following are ototoxic agents **EXCEPT**
- **A.** chloroquine
- **B.** salicylates
- **C.** ampicillin
- **D.** nicotine
- **E.** caffeine

**623.** The main delayed effect of ionizing radiation is
- **A.** carcinogenesis
- **B.** pulmonary fibrosis
- **C.** endocarditis
- **D.** decreased WBC count
- **E.** dermatitis

**624.** The most important cellular target for ionizing radiation is
A. mitochondria
B. DNA
C. endoplasmic reticulum
D. cell wall
E. lysosome

**625.** The earliest effects of ionizing radiation are seen in
A. elevated sedimentation rate
B. lymphocyte count reduction
C. lymphocyte count proliferation
D. decreased RBC count
E. change in RBC size and shape

**626.** The most common source of ionizing radiation exposure is
A. x-rays
B. cosmic rays
C. ground
D. lightning
E. television

**627.** Which one of the following applies to nonionizing radiation?
A. Energy value of electromagnetic radiation is less than ionizing radiation
B. Wavelength is shorter than that of ionizing radiation
C. Effect of radiation doesn't depend on the duration of exposure
D. Is not produced by the sun
E. Has no carcinogenic risk

**628.** In reference to UV radiation, all of the following are true **EXCEPT**
A. the sun is the major source of UV radiation
B. the amount of UV radiation varies with season, time of day, and altitude
C. dark clothing filters out UV radiation efficiently
D. it has an important role in the prevention of rickets
E. certain suntan lotions can effectively protect the skin

**629.** Excessive exposure to natural and man-made sources of infrared radiation cause adverse health effects mainly to the
   A. lymphatic system
   B. gonads
   C. nervous system
   D. eyes and skin
   E. immune system

**630.** Several epidemiologic studies have found the most predictive indicator of at risk populations for malignant melanoma is
   A. cumulative childhood exposure to UV light
   B. frequency of childhood sunburns
   C. amount of pigmentation of the skin
   D. sun exposure as an adult
   E. living in proximity to the equator

**631.** All of the following about infrared radiation are true **EXCEPT**
   A. can burn the skin
   B. can cause cataract development
   C. has a longer wavelength than visible light
   D. is primary radiation in "tanning booths"
   E. is a potential health hazard to glassblowers

**632.** Extremely low-frequency (ELF) electromagnetic field is
   A. associated with electronic office equipment and home appliances
   B. a possible cause of retinal and testicular cancer
   C. a side product of x-rays
   D. unable to cause biologic changes
   E. an apparent factor in the development of psychoses

# Environmental Health Issues

## Answers and Discussion

**476.** (C)   Radon exposure is very common because of its widespread occurrence. It is naturally released from the ground and contaminates many houses, especially those with basements. Estimates range from 5000 to 20,000 lung cancer deaths per year as a result of radon exposure. (**Ref. 5,** pp. 503, 505)

**477.** (C)   Mercury poisoning can cause tremors and ataxia. It may also cause emotional lability, neurasthesias, and psychomotor disturbances. Organic mercury can cause visual field changes, while inorganic mercury can produce personality disturbances. (**Ref. 5,** pp. 268–272)

**478.** (B)   Asbestosis can occur in family members of people who worked with asbestos. Also, asbestosis may continue progression long after exposure ends, because of the durability of the fibers and their ability to continue to stimulate macrophages for years without being degraded. Chest roentgenogram findings in asbestosis typically show irregular opacities in the lower lung fields. Pleural thickening often occurs, but not always. (**Ref. 2,** pp. 350, 351; **Ref. 77,** p. 2339)

**479.** (C)   When asbestosis is present but not severe enough to directly cause acute asbestosis and premature death, the most likely related cause of mortality is lung cancer. (**Ref. 2,** pp. 356–359)

**480. (A)** Asbestos causes pulmonary fibrosis when macrophages phagocytize fibrils, then release factors such as fibronectin, which stimulate fibroblasts to proliferate and produce collagen. Asbestos fibrils do migrate to the pleura and can also cause pleural fibrosis. The answers C and D are also correct, but they are unrelated to pulmonary fibrosis. (**Ref. 2,** pp. 348, 349)

**481. (A)** For asbestosis, there is decreased $FEV_1$ (obstructive disease) and increased residual volume, with the TLC remaining the same or even increasing slightly. However, the residual volume (RV):TLC ratio increases, and the vital capacity decreases. This does not necessarily indicate restrictive disease, however, since it may be due only to the increased RV. (**Ref. 2,** p. 353; **Ref. 77,** p. 2339)

**482. (B)** For complicated coal worker's pneumoconiosis (also called progressive massive fibrosis), there is decreased $FEV_1$ (obstructive disease) and decreased TLC (restrictive disease). There may also be an increase in residual volume. (**Ref. 77,** p. 2338)

**483. (D)** Coal worker's pneumoconiosis has two forms, simple and complicated (which is also called progressive massive fibrosis [PMF]). Symptoms do not usually occur in nonsmokers until PMF develops. In this case, there will be a background of small rounded opacities (which are seen early), generally with at least one shadow over 1 cm in diameter. Subsequently, as the disease progresses, large conglomerate shadows may be seen. (**Ref. 2,** pp. 358–365; **Ref. 77,** p. 2338)

**484. (D)** Coal worker's pneumoconiosis puts people at increased risk of developing *Mycobacterium tuberculosis* infection. It does not increase risk of the other diseases mentioned. (**Ref. 2,** p. 368)

**485. (B)** Coal worker's pneumoconiosis increases risk of gastric cancer, through compounds in the coal undergoing nitrosation or interacting with other chemicals to form carcinogenic substances. It does not increase the risk of the other cancers listed. (**Ref. 2,** p. 368)

**486. (B)** Long-term inhalation of chromium compounds in chromium-plating workshops has caused severe corrosion of the nasal mucous membranes, often resulting in a defect in the septum. The ulcer is not painful, but bleeding and sneezing often occur. Irritation of airways, cornea, and conjunctiva may result. Chromium may cause circumscribed ulcers (chrome holes) at the knuckles, nail roots, or other exposed skin areas. Even though they may be quite deep, they are almost painless. (**Ref. 2,** p. 387)

**487. (B)** Chromium is one of the best-known allergens in the occupational environment, and chromate is frequently the most common cause of allergic contact dermatitis among men. Chromium is a well-documented human carcinogen, and occupational exposures from the production of chromates, chromium pigments, and perhaps ferrochrome, have caused an increased frequency of cancer in the respiratory tract. (**Ref. 2,** p. 387)

**488. (D)** Iron is necessary for life but is toxic at excess exposures. Iron deficiency is the most prevalent metal deficiency syndrome in humans, especially among women in the reproductive age group and certain groups of small children. (**Ref. 2,** p. 389)

**489. (D)** Ingestion of iron supplements in considerable excess may cause acute gastrointestinal lesions followed by metabolic acidosis, toxic hepatitis, and shock. Chronic iron overload leads to hemosiderosis and liver cirrhosis. Foundry workers, grinders, and welders are exposed to considerable quantities of iron oxide fumes, which accumulate in the lungs and may result in siderosis, a benign and reversible pneumoconiosis. (**Ref. 2,** p. 389)

**490. (C)** Of clinical importance are the chronic effects of lead on the red blood cells and the nervous system. Anemia is a typical symptom in classic lead poisoning. Lead inhibits the Na-K-ATPase in the cell membrane of the erythrocytes, making them less stable and thus shortening their life-span. Lead affects both the central and peripheral nervous systems. In the past, acute toxic encephalopathy occurred in relation to severe lead exposure in certain occupations. More recently, cases in adults have been associated with consumption of moonshine whiskey distilled in old car radiators. Children are more susceptible to central nervous system effects, sometimes as a result of ingesting paint flakes containing lead from peeling walls. (**Ref. 2,** p. 390)

**491. (A)** Acute mercury vapor poisoning causes severe airway irritation, chemical pneumonitis, and pulmonary edema. Tremor may indicate nervous system involvement, but pulmonary distress is usually the cause of death. Ingestion of inorganic compounds results in symptoms of gastrointestinal corrosion and irritation such as vomiting, bloody diarrhea, and stomach pains. Shock and acute kidney dysfunction with uremia may ensue. (**Ref. 2, p.** 393)

492. **(B)** Until recently, radon was regarded as a health hazard only for uranium miners. Radon is dangerous because it is radioactive, undergoing decay to produce a series of radon daughters. These can be inhaled and deposited in the lungs, where they constitute an internal source of alpha radiation exposure, increasing the risk of lung cancer. The Environmental Protection Agency estimates that between 7000 and 30,000 lung cancer deaths each year are caused by indoor radon exposure. (**Ref. 5, p.** 505)

493. **(B)** Nickel allergy is the most frequent cause of contact allergy in women. The development of allergy is frequently provoked by earrings, but metal buttons, bracelets, and watches are also frequent causes. Some studies suggest that about 10% to 15% of women become allergic to nickel and that almost half of them at some point develop hand eczema, in some cases so severe that the patient has to stop working. (**Ref. 2, p.** 395)

494. **(A)** Occupational lead exposure occurs in particular in the following processes: primary production of lead from lead ores, secondary lead production from used automobile batteries and scrap metal; production of batteries; welding and lead cutting of flame containing or minimum treated alloys; molding of lead-containing alloys in foundries; soldering with lead solder if the temperature is too high; grinding and sandblasting of lead alloys and coatings. Research has shown insidious effects that produce a chronic toxic encephalopathy in adults. Typically the patient is taken to the physician or the hospital by the wife, who is worried by his failing health and his unbearable irritability. Chemical examination and neuropsychologic testing frequently show that attention, concentration, memory, and abstraction are affected. (**Ref. 2, pp.** 389, 390)

495. **(D)** Anemia is typical in classic lead poisoning. Lead inhibits the Na-K-ATPase in cell membranes of the erythrocytes, making them less stable and thereby shortening their life-span. (**Ref. 2, p.** 390)

**496. (A)** Asbestos exposure causes excessive death rates not only for lung cancer, mesothelioma, and asbestosis, but also for cancers of the gastrointestinal tract, larynx, oropharynx, and kidney. Lung cancer, either squamous cell or adenocarcinoma, is the most frequent cancer associated with asbestos exposure. Mesotheliomas are also associated with asbestos but do not seem to be increased with smoking. (**Ref. 2,** p. 344)

**497. (E)** Carbon tetrachloride causes hepatoxicity, both clinically and in various experimental models. Hepatocellular carcinoma has also been reported to occur several years after carbon tetrachloride poisoning. (**Ref. 2,** p. 411)

**498. (A)** See answer 496 above.

**499. (D)** Leukemia secondary to benzene exposure has been repeatedly reported since the 1930s. All types of leukemia have been found. Malignant transformation of the bone marrow has been noted years after cessation of exposure. (**Ref. 2,** p. 408)

**500. (B)** Mercury damages both the peripheral and the central nervous systems. The fine-intention tremor of the fingers, eyelids, lips, and tongue may progress to spasms of the arms and legs. Central nervous system effects include restlessness, irritability, insomnia, concentration difficulties, decreased memory, and depression. (**Ref. 2,** p. 393)

**501. (C)** Silicosis is a fibrotic lung disease produced by the inhalation of dust containing free crystalline silicon dioxide. Silicotic nodules are readily felt in the lung and on the cut surface, measuring between 2 and 6 mm, located more frequently in the apical and posterior part of the lung. (**Ref. 2,** p. 374)

**502. (A)** Lead is found throughout the environment in soils, water, air, and food. With the exception of occupational exposures to lead, the major source of lead intake is through drinking water, ie, tap water from lead pipes or lead solder in household plumbing. Leafy vegetables or fruits are a significant source of lead exposure, sometimes showing as much as 3000 ppm, particularly if grown in gardens near busy freeways. Canned foods, if they are in lead-soldered cans, are also a significant source of lead. Milk is rarely mentioned as a significant source. (**Ref. 5,** pp. 258, 260)

**503.** (**B**)   Radon is a colorless, odorless radioactive gas that may cause between 7000 and 30,000 lung cancer deaths a year. Radon occurs naturally in the environment when underground radium decays. The radioactive gas seeps toward the surface and can enter homes through faulty pipe seals or cracks in walls. (**Ref. 5,** pp. 503–506)

**504.** (**B**)   Ethylene glycol is a viscous colorless liquid, used mainly in antifreeze and hydraulic fluids. Hemodialysis has been successful in the treatment of accidental ethylene glycol poisoning by ingestion. The most important preventive action is to alert employees to the extreme hazard of ingestion. (**Ref. 2,** p. 419)

**505.** (**B**)   Contrary to common fears, swallowing inorganic mercury, such as would occur if an oral thermometer were to break while in the mouth, poses virtually no health threat. Such mercury simply passes through the gastrointestinal tract and is excreted through the kidneys in a few days. (**Ref. 5,** pp. 268–272)

**506.** (**E**)   Lead inhibits the Na-K-ATPase in the cell membranes of the erythrocytes as well as other steps in the formation of heme, leading to anemia. Direct axonal damage also occurs, leading to peripheral and central nervous system defects. In severe poisoning, colicky pains occur as a result of cramps in the smooth muscle of the intestines. (**Ref. 2,** p. 390)

**507.** (**D**)   Pralidoxime can reactivate cholinesterase if given within 24 to 48 hours of poisoning. (**Ref. 2,** pp. 481, 482)

**508.** (**C**)   Chlorinated hydrocarbons are CNS stimulants, highly lipophilic, biodegrade slowly, and can cause anxiety, tremor, hyperexcitability, and generalized seizures. (**Ref. 2,** pp. 482, 483)

**509.** (**A**)   High mortality with paraquat is associated with ingestion, accidental or in a suicide attempt. Paraquat causes damage to the liver, kidney, and myocardium. However, relentless pulmonary fibrosis is the usual mechanism causing death. (**Ref. 2,** pp. 483, 484)

**510. (D)** Signs of fumigant intoxication include pulmonary edema (the most frequent cause of death), neurotoxicity, and behavioral effects including toxic psychosis. (**Ref. 2,** pp. 484, 485)

**511. (C)** Pesticides cause the following cancers: non-Hodgkin's lymphoma, leukemia, multiple myeloma, liver cancer, brain cancer, and lung cancer. (**Ref. 2,** p. 485)

**512. (D)** Major factors affecting thermoregulation include heat production by metabolism, heat loss by evaporation, heat loss or gain by convection, and heat loss or gain by radiation. (**Ref. 2,** p. 492)

**513. (B)** Heat stroke is the most serious illness caused by elevated temperature. The core body temperature is elevated to greater than 105°F. Mental status is altered, while sweating can be profuse or absent. The treatment is directed toward the rapid lowering of body temperature. (**Ref. 2,** p. 493)

**514. (C)** Heat exhaustion is caused by the unbalanced or inadequate replacement of water and salts lost in perspiration resulting from thermal stress. It usually develops in several days, body temperature may be normal or moderately elevated, symptoms are primarily weakness and treatment is supportive. (**Ref. 2,** p. 493)

**515. (A)** Heat syncope is a transient fall in blood pressure with an associated loss of consciousness. Prevention is by avoiding strenuous exercise in heat. It occurs secondary to transient fluid and electrolyte abnormalities. (**Ref. 2,** p. 493)

**516. (C)** Persons at risk for heat-related illness are the elderly, infants and children, and urban dwellers. The death rate is greater in men than women and in the obese than nonobese. Also, a previous history of heat stroke puts a person at greater risk. (**Ref. 2,** p. 494)

**517. (E)** Surveillance for occupational disease and injury has three basic components: (1) the detection and enumeration of occupationally related morbidity and mortality; (2) data evaluation and interpretation to characterize trends and identify clusters of disease and injury; (3) intervention to decrease the incidence or severity of occupational disease and injury in data collection and analysis. (**Ref. 2,** p. 551)

**518. (E)** Surveillance activities include medical screening, medical monitoring, biologic monitoring, and exposure monitoring. **(Ref. 2, p. 551)**

**519. (A)** According to the National Institute for Occupational Safety and Health (NIOSH) list of leading causes of work-related diseases, occupational lung disease is number one. **(Ref. 2, p. 552, Table 31–1)**

**520. (E)** The ten leading causes of work-related illness include disorders of reproduction, severe occupational traumatic injuries (amputations), noise-induced hearing loss, and skin disorders. **(Ref. 2, p. 552, Table 31–1)**

**521. (D)** Neurotoxic disorders include peripheral neuropathy, toxic encephalitis, psychoses, and extreme personality changes. **(Ref. 2, p. 552)**

**522. (A)** Medical screening is defined as testing to diagnose disease in individuals at an early and hopefully reversible stage. **(Ref. 2, p. 551)**

**523. (C)** The Rehabilitation Act enacted in 1973 prohibits the federal government from discriminating against a person based on a handicap (mental or physical impairment). **(Ref. 2, p. 561)**

**524. (C)** Estimates from the United States National Health Survey show 11.5% of the United States working age population are disabled. **(Ref. 2, p. 560)**

**525. (B)** African-Americans and Latino-Americans have more disabilities when compared to whites. **(Ref. 2, p. 560)**

**526. (E)** Compared with persons in the 25- to 34-year-old age group, 55- to 64-year-olds are four times more likely to be work disabled. The 55- to 64-year-old age group has the highest likelihood of disabilities compared with the other listed age groups. **(Ref. 2, p. 560)**

**527. (A)** Low income correlates inversely with disability. **(Ref. 2, p. 560)**

**528. (A)** There is a strong correlation between low educational level and disability (inverse relationship). **(Ref. 2,** p. 560)

**529. (A)** Conducting a job analysis is the first step in a rational assessment of any individual's ability to perform required job tasks. **(Ref. 2,** p. 560)

**530. (B)** Diarrhea, weakness, headaches, and listlessness can be observed in those with acute pesticide exposure. **(Ref. 2,** p. 566)

**531. (D)** California is the only state that mandates physician reporting of pesticide-related illness. **(Ref. 2,** p. 566)

**532. (A)** Dermatitis is the foremost work-related health problem in agriculture. **(Ref. 2,** p. 567)

**533. (C)** Inadequate sanitation leads to increase risk of communicable diseases, heat stress, urinary tract infections, and pesticide-related illnesses. **(Ref. 2,** p. 567)

**534. (A)** The higher incidence of cancer is probably due to numerous lifestyle factors, including alcohol consumption and tobacco use and sexually transmitted diseases. **(Ref. 2,** p. 813)

**535. (C)** Noise can interfere with a child's ability to distinguish certain sounds and thus may adversely affect language development. In addition, hearing loss, teratogenesis, and decreased work performance can be caused by noise. **(Ref. 5,** p. 533)

**536. (A)** Noise-induced hearing loss is usually preceded by tinnitus. **(Ref. 5,** p. 527)

**537. (E)** Prevention of noise-induced hearing loss includes reducing the noise in the workplace, ear protection (ear defenders), and special equipment that has noise restriction implementation. **(Ref. 2,** pp. 528, 529)

**538. (A)** 300 to 4000 Hz. **(Ref. 5,** p. 521)

**539. (A)** The definition of sociocucus is hearing loss as a result of loud noises. **(Ref. 5,** p. 527)

**540.** **(C)** Presbycusis is hearing loss resulting from old age. (**Ref. 5,** p. 527)

**541.** **(D)** Temporary threshold shift is a partial hearing loss that occurs after sudden exposure to a loud noise. It usually last a few hours, but hearing loss can be permanent. (**Ref. 5,** p. 528)

**542.** **(D)** OSHA does require employers to keep health and safety records. (**Ref. 2,** p. 547)

**543.** **(B)** NIOSH is the principal federal agency engaged in research to eliminate on-the-job hazards to the health and safety of American workers. NIOSH has a training grant program to develop baccalaureate and graduate programs in colleges and universities. (**Ref. 2,** p. 548)

**544.** **(D); 545. (C); 546. (A); 547. (B)** The Food and Agriculture Organization (FAO) and World Health Organization (WHO) of the United Nations created the Codex Alimentarius Commission to implement a food standards program, to protect the health of consumers, and to ensure fair practice in world trade, coordination of food standards, activity of international organizations, form food standards, and publicize accepted standards. The FDA is the federal agency in the United States ensuring food safety. Occupational Safety and Health Administration (OSHA) is responsible for all working conditions and the United States Department of Agriculture (USDA) inspects agricultural products in the United States. (**Ref. 2,** p. 592)

**548.** **(B)** Bacterial agents are responsible for the majority of outbreaks of food-borne illness. (**Ref. 2,** p. 590)

**549.** **(A)** *Staphylococcus aureus* causes food-borne intoxication and has a heat-stable enterotoxin. The severity of illness depends on the amount of the enterotoxin ingested. *Salmonella, Campylobacter,* and *Listeria* produce food-borne infection. (**Ref. 2,** pp. 590–592)

**550.** **(D)** The great majority of incidents of botulism have been associated with home-canned vegetables in the United States. In the former Soviet Union, Canada, and Japan most outbreaks are associated with fish or fish products. Pork is the most common vehicle for staphylococcus infection. Rice has been associated with *Bacillus cereus* intoxication. (**Ref. 2,** pp. 590–592)

**551.** (**B**)   The etiologic agents most often responsible for food-borne disease in the United States have been *Salmonella* species, *Staphylococcus aureus,* and *Clostridium perfringens. Salmonella* species is the most frequently confirmed causative agent. *Campylobacter* is considered the most frequent cause of bacterial diarrhea in the United States. (**Ref. 2,** pp. 590, 592)

**552.** (**C**)   Fruits and vegetables require storage at desired temperatures and relative humidity to prevent deterioration and maintain freshness. The storage facility must be kept under sanitary conditions to protect grain from rodent and insect infestation. Grains that are dried before storage then require protection from moisture to prevent the growth of mold. Irradiation has become an acceptable alternative to ethylene bromide, which is an insecticide no longer permitted for food application. (**Ref. 2,** p. 594)

**553.** (**D**)   *Campylobacter, Listeria, Staphylococcus, Brucella, Yersinia,* and *Salmonella* are associated with contaminated raw milk. *Staphylococcus* is often associated with clinical or subclinical mastitis. If raw milk is not rapidly chilled, staphylococci grow and produce enterotoxin. Milk should be cooled to 7°C within 2 hours after milking. (**Ref. 2,** pp. 595, 596)

**554.** (**C**)   Sanitizing equipment involves heat at 93°C for 5 to 30 minutes. This method is often not economical in food processing plants because of heating and cooling costs and is generally used in small-scale food handling operations. Ultraviolet radiation sanitizes nonporous surfaces and water. Some of the major types of chemical sanitizing agents are chlorine and iodine compounds. (**Ref. 2,** pp. 600, 601)

**555.** (**B**)   Freezing to minus 10°C results in complete inhibition of bacterial growth. Dehydration inactivates many food pathogens; however *Salmonella, Listeria,* and *Staphylococcus* can be expected to survive in stored dried foods. Refrigeration delays deterioration, but cold-tolerant bacteria, including *Listeria monocytogenes, Clostridium botulinum* type E, and *Yersinia enterocolitica* will grow in a home refrigerator set at 4° to 7°C. Blanching can reduce microbial content by up to 99% but is not a reliable method of bacterial growth inhibition. (**Ref. 2,** pp. 603–606)

**556.** (**A**)   Unsafe time–temperature relationships occur in transport, storage preparation, cooking service, and post cooking storage of food. (**Ref. 2,** pp. 609–611)

**557.** (**B**)   Meats including pork, ham, chicken, turkey , beef, and milk products, baked goods, and mixed salads are associated with staphylococcus intoxication. Pork, especially ham that is prepared whole, is difficult to cool rapidly and thoroughly reheat. (**Ref. 2,** pp. 590, 591)

**558.** (**D**); **559.** (**C**); **560.** (**A**); **561.** (**B**)   Pasteurized Grade A Milk Ordinance (PMO) revised in 1978 regulates milk production, transportation, and processing. The Codex Alimentarius Commission was created by the WHO and FAO to protect the health of consumers, ensure fair practice in world trade, form food standards, publish food standards, and promote coordination of food standards of international organizations. The Delaney clause is in the Food Additives Amendment. It prohibits approval of any substance as a food additive that has been found to cause cancer in humans or animals. The GRAS (Generally Recognized As Safe) list is a list of food additives that was exempt from regulation by the Food Additives Amendment (1958), with substances found to be of questionable safety being removed from the list. (**Ref. 2,** pp. 589, 592, 593)

**562.** (**B**)   The average per capita consumption of water in a typical American community is 600 liters a day. Forty percent of water is used for toilet flushing, 30% for bathing, 15% for laundry, 5% for drinking and cooking, and 5% for dishwashing. In Asia the per capita consumption of water may be only 50 liters a day. (**Ref. 2,** pp. 619, 620)

**563.** (**D**)   Groundwater recharges through percolation of rainwater and runoff into the soil. It tends to be more mineralized than surface water. It generally has higher sanitary quality and is not nearly as subject to pollution as surface water. Passage of rainwater through the soil serves to improve its bacteriologic quality, although groundwater polluted from toxic waste discharge and landfill has become a major problem in some areas. Surface water stored in a lake provides opportunity for coagulation and sedimentation of colloidal suspended solids. (**Ref. 2,** pp. 620–623)

**564.** (C) Rainwater is the primary source of fresh water. (**Ref. 2,** p. 621)

**565.** (C) There is approximately 1500 million cubic kilometers of water in the world. Only about 0.2% of this is fresh water readily available for use. (**Ref. 2,** p. 619)

**566.** (C) Storage provides the opportunity for coagulation and sedimentation of colloids and suspended solid particles; exposure to sunlight may provide some measure of disinfection; and a large body of water can attenuate high levels of contaminants, such as spills from tankers. Accumulation of nutrients occurs, especially in standing water such as lakes, may cause eutrophication. (**Ref. 2,** pp. 621, 622)

**567.** (D) Inhalation of fibers has been associated with peritoneal mesothelioma, pleural plaques, and lung cancer. Ingestion of asbestos through drinking water has been associated with an excess risk of gastrointestinal tract cancers. (**Ref. 2,** p. 628)

**568.** (B) Radon is a naturally occurring radionucleide in groundwater. Seventy percent of groundwater supplies have detectable radon concentrations. (**Ref. 2,** p. 628)

**569.** (B) *Cryptosporidium,* adenovirus, hepatitis A virus, and polio virus cause water-borne diseases by ingestion. Schistosomiasis is caused by larval migration through the skin. (**Ref. 2,** p. 630)

**570.** (B) Disinfection with chlorine has been the most important process for assuring safety of potable water with reference to bacteria. Water-borne infections that have occurred have generally been traced back to failure in chlorination. Filtration, iodine, and sedimentation are other methods used in water purification. (**Ref. 2,** pp. 632–637)

**571.** (A) Copper sulfate may be used for algae control in lakes and reservoirs. The copper ions are algicidal but not bactericidal. Silver ions are bactericidal although their action is slow. Mercury vapor arc lamps and irradiation with ultraviolet light are also methods of disinfection. Ferric salts are used as coagulants in water purification. (**Ref. 2,** pp. 633, 635)

**572. (C)** Biochemical oxygen demand measures the oxygen requirements of bacteria and other organisms as they feed on and decompose organic matter. This determines whether the body of water remains aerobic or anaerobic. Chemical oxygen demand and total organic carbon determination are useful indicators of water quality where industrial wastes are present. (**Ref. 2,** p. 641)

**573. (C); 574. (A); 575. (B); 576. (D)** Sulfates in drinking water can have a laxative effect; the effect is more pronounced in occasional users. Methemoglobinemia has occurred in infants after ingestion of well water containing high levels of nitrates. There is an inverse relationship between hard water and cardiovascular disease mortality rate. Softening of water by ion exchange adds significant concentrations of sodium to the water. (**Ref. 2,** pp. 627, 628, 629)

**577. (C)** Safe distances of a privy from a well depend on numerous factors. These include: height and direction of groundwater flow, the nature of the soil, and distance from groundwater. No safe distance can be prescribed when the privy is in limestone or a similar geologic formation. (**Ref. 2,** p. 639)

**578. (B)** Chlorine in waste-water treatment used where effluents are to be discharged to waters used for shellfish growing, drinking, or bathing. Chlorination can result in chloramine formation, which may be toxic to aquatic life. Chlorinated hydrocarbons may be formed. Destruction of beneficial microorganisms, as well as pathogens, may occur. (**Ref. 2,** p. 644)

**579. (C)** Reclamation of waste water has been used for irrigation, industry (process and cooling), recreation in lakes and ponds, and nonpotable residential and commercial use. Reclamation for potable purposes is not recommended. (**Ref. 2,** p. 647)

**580. (B)** Solid waste disposal methods are incineration and landfill. Landfill disposal is the dominant form of solid waste disposal in the United States. Recycling and composting are material recovery from solid waste. (**Ref. 2,** p. 649)

**581. (B)** Incineration is used in Japan and some European countries. It stabilizes and eliminates hazardous materials, turns organic to inorganic material, kills pathogens, and reduces waste quantity down to one fifteenth to one twentieth of the volume. Over time waste that is disposed underground, as in landfills, will cause ground subsidence. (**Ref. 2,** pp. 650, 651)

**582. (B)** Municipal solid waste contains a high quantity of plastic waste, which is high in chlorides. Chlorides produce hydrogen chloride gas when incinerated. The sulfur content in municipal waste is generally low. (**Ref. 2,** p. 655)

**583. (D); 584. (B); 585. (C); 586. (A)** In material recovery and recycling, resource recovery with and without property conversion of the recycled waste is used. Aluminum cans are transformed into raw material for remanufacture and glass bottles are cleaned, sterilized, and reused as new. The use of kitchen garbage to prepare compost is an example of resource recovery with conversion of the recovered material. The energy released in the incineration of combustible and nonhazardous waste can be used as thermal electromotive energy. (**Ref. 2,** p. 656)

**587. (C)** The most important exposure pathway from radioactive waste disposal is groundwater. (**Ref. 2,** p. 659)

**588. (B)** Ozone attains the maximum density at an altitude of approximately 22 km. It is present at measurable concentrations at 10 to 35 km. (**Ref. 2,** p. 662)

**589. (D)** As one ascends in altitude, the density of air decreases exponentially. (**Ref. 2,** p. 662)

**590. (E)** Hypoxia is particularly dangerous because it produces little discomfort. Subtle symptoms at altitudes of 2000 to 3000 m include drowsiness, difficulty with night vision, slow thinking, difficulty with calculations, and delayed reaction time. (**Ref. 2,** p. 663)

**591. (B)** The processing of visual information is influenced by the vestibular system and to some extent by proprioception and motion. The vision sensory system is the most important modality for maintenance of our spatial orientation. The interaction between vision and vestibular function is important in the fine tuning of our spatial orientation. **(Ref. 2,** p. 664)

**592. (C)** The earth's atmosphere shields us from the potential dangers of space radiation. The duration of exposure is much more prolonged in space. **(Ref. 2,** p. 664)

**593. (C)** Biomedical challenges associated with short-duration space flights include space motion sickness, cardiovascular deconditioning, bone mineral loss, and loss of red cell mass. **(Ref. 2,** p. 665)

**594. (C)** The lowest blood alcohol level that has been found to adversely compromise flight performance is 0.04% (40 mg/dL). **(Ref. 2,** p. 667)

**595. (C)** The most prevalent indoor environment in the world is huts in rural communities of developing countries. **(Ref. 2,** p. 671)

**596. (C)** In developing countries indoor air pollution from biomass fuel combustion is a difficult problem. Premature death from chronic obstructive pulmonary disease is common among women who from childhood have been exposed to fumes from primitive cooking stoves. **(Ref. 2,** p. 672)

**597. (E)** Rats exposed to formaldehyde have demonstrated an increased risk of nasopharyngeal cancer. Urea-formaldehyde foam insulation has been banned in many areas on the basis of the evidence that it is associated with carcinogenicity in rats. **(Ref. 2,** p. 672)

**598. (B); 599. (C); 600. (B); 601. (A)** Studies have shown the association between mental health disorders and urban living conditions. Schizophrenia and alcoholism have maximum prevalence in slums and skid row districts. Depression is clustered in neighborhoods where a high proportion of the people live in single-room rented apartments. Adolescent delinquency, vandalism, and underachievement at school have a high prevalence in dormitory suburbs occupied by low-paid workers. (**Ref. 2,** p. 673)

**602.** **(C)** Carbon dioxide, oxides of nitrogen, methane, chlorofluorocarbons, and ozone are associated with the greenhouse effect. (**Ref. 2,** p. 677)

**603.** **(B)** Sources of methane include agriculture and rotting vegetation. At high latitudes, warming as a result of the greenhouse effect could thaw the permafrost and release frozen rotting vegetation in arctic bogs and ponds, emitting large amounts of methane and contributing to atmospheric greenhouse gases. (**Ref. 2,** pp. 677, 678)

**604.** **(D)** An important adverse effect of ozone depletion is its effect on single celled and small organisms, especially plankton in the surface waters of the oceans, since these are the beginning of many food chains. (**Ref. 2,** p. 679)

**605.** **(B)** The principal pathologic lesions caused by the presence of asbestos in the lungs involve the membranous and respiratory bronchioles. These lesions physically narrow these small airways and limit mid and terminal flow rates, that is, obstruct expiratory airflow as the earliest physiologic lesion in asbestosis. It appears that the obstruction of the small airways occurs before the irregular opacities of asbestosis are visible on the chest roentgenogram. (**Ref. 2,** p. 353)

**606.** **(C)** The profusion of irregular opacities on the chest radiograph is used as the anatomic measure of severity of asbestosis, and key pulmonary function measurements are plotted against this anatomic score. Progressive impairment of airflow and air trapping is seen with an increasing profusion of opacities on radiographs. (**Ref. 2,** p. 353)

**607.** **(A)** The major public health concern and principal cause of death from asbestosis in developed countries is lung cancer. In some groups of asbestos-exposed workers, the lung cancer mortality rate is as high as one in five. The cocausality with cigarette smoking is clear, and the relative risk may be 50 to 100 times as high in the asbestos-exposed smoker as in the non–asbestos-exposed subject who has never smoked. (**Ref. 2,** p. 356)

**608. (B)** The key to preventing coal worker's pneumoconiosis is prevention of prolonged inhalation of significant concentrations of coal dust. This can be accomplished in two ways: (1) by the control of respirable coal-mine dust through proper ventilation of mining operations, or (2) by removal of miners with early evidence of CWP to low-dust jobs. Of these two, dust control is more effective. **(Ref. 2, p. 369)**

**609. (E)** There are no pathognomonic signs or symptoms of CWP. In the early stages of the disease, workers frequently are asymptomatic and without functional impairment. Chronic cough and phlegm are, however, associated with prolonged inhalation of coal dust and with cigarette smoking. These symptoms per se are not necessarily associated with functional impairment. **(Ref. 2, p. 368)**

**610. (C)** **(Ref. 2, p. 366)**

**611. (A)** The FDA regulates bottled water; the Clean Water Act requires fishable swimmable waters; only the Safe Drinking Water Act requires the EPA to set MCLs. **(Ref. 90, pp. 480–481)**

**612. (D)** The Hazard Communication has three major areas of emphasis: maintenance of materials safety data sheets, labeling, and appropriate training. **(Ref. 90, p. 750)**

**613. (C)** Secondary standards are meant to protect livestock, crops, and structures. **(Ref. 90, pp. 745, 746)**

**614. (B)** Enforcement activities are conducted by OSHA; NIOSH conducts research; AIHA and OSHRC and ACGIH do not conduct inspections. **(Ref. 90, p. 750)**

**615. (E)** TSCA requires manufacturers to test substances, report test results to the EPA, and empowers EPA to remove suspect substances from the marketplace. In addition, it regulates use and disposal of hazardous substances. **(Ref. 90, p. 750)**

**616. (A)** Methylene chloride is metabolized to carbon monoxide, which subsequently increases carboxyhemoglobin concentrations. **(Ref. 91, p. 445)**

**617. (D)** Lipid solubility, molecular weight, and polarity all play an important role in the ability of toxic substances to passively transfer from plasma to breast milk. (**Ref. 91,** p. 486)

**618. (C)** Hepatitis B is the most frequent work-related infectious disease in the United States. (**Ref. 91,** pp. 281–286)

**619. (C)** Hearing loss first becomes apparent in audiometric examinations in the 4000-Hz range. (**Ref. 91,** pp. 254–257)

**620. (C)** Conductive hearing loss is usually associated with interferences of sound transmission in the outer or middle ear. Examples include damage to the footplate of the stapes, as in otosclerosis, or the mobility of the eardrum and ossicle caused by fluid. (**Ref. 90,** p. 252)

**621. (B)** Cumulative hair cell damage on the organ of Corti results in hearing loss. (**Ref. 91,** pp. 250–254)

**622. (E)** Many common chemicals and drugs are considered ototoxic agents. (**Ref. 90,** p. 254)

**623. (A)** Although pulmonary fibrosis, endocarditis, and decreased WBC count can occur with exposure to ionizing radiation, the main *delayed* effect is carcinogenesis. (**Ref. 2,** p. 506)

**624. (B)** DNA is the most important target for ionizing radiation. (**Ref. 2,** p. 503)

**625. (B)** Lymphocyte count reduction, not proliferation, is the earliest effect of ionizing radiation. Decreased RBC count and elevated sedimentation rate are not seen with ionizing radiation. (**Ref. 2,** p. 504)

**626. (C)** The most common form of radiation is from radon, which is found in igneous rock. (**Ref. 2,** p. 509)

**627. (A)** Nonionizing radiation has less energy value than ionizing radiation, is emitted from the sun, can contribute to skin cancer, and its effect is dependent on the duration of exposure. Nonionizing radiation wavelength is longer than that of ionizing radiation. (**Ref. 2,** p. 513)

**628. (C)** Dark clothing can filter out some UV radiation, but not efficiently. The sun is the major source of UV radiation, and the amount someone is exposed to does vary with time of day, altitude, and season. UV radiation has an important role in preventing rickets via photoproduction of vitamin D in the skin. (**Ref. 2,** pp. 513, 514)

**629. (D)** The iris and cornea are particularly susceptible to infrared exposure. Effects to the skin include capillary bed vasodilation and increased pigmentation. (**Ref. 2,** p. 518)

**630. (B)** Frequency of childhood sunburns are the most predictive indicator of at-risk populations for malignant melanoma. (**Ref. 2,** p. 514)

**631. (D)** Infrared radiation can burn the skin, cause cataract development, has a longer wavelength than visible light, and is a potential health hazard to glassblowers. Ultraviolet light is the primary emission of tanning booth light bulbs. (**Ref. 2,** p. 518)

**632. (A)** ELF is radiation in 0- to 300-Hz frequencies, and exposure is commonly electronic office equipment and home appliances. There have been links between these fields and childhood cancers (leukemia and brain tumors), breast cancer, and depression. (**Ref. 2,** p. 518)

# 5

# Health Care Organization

**633.** A systems approach to health care emphasizes the interdependencies among the parts of the system and between the organizational assets and finances. Essential participants in decision making in the health care system include each of the following **EXCEPT**
- **A.** provider
- **B.** consumer
- **C.** policy maker
- **D.** payer
- **E.** dependents

**634.** All of the following changes have influenced the function of the American health care system significantly **EXCEPT**
- **A.** the demographic composition of the United States
- **B.** the nature of disease
- **C.** improved technology
- **D.** availability of providers
- **E.** medicolegal issues

**635.** Which of the following was in the top five causes of death in both 1900 and 1985?
- **A.** Heart disease
- **B.** Tuberculosis

C. Accidents
D. Cancer
E. Diabetes

636. The ultimate source of authority within the organizational structure of a hospital is
A. the administration
B. the medical staff
C. the governing board
D. the peer review board
E. the institutional review board

637. Group medical practices have grown in response to each of the following factors **EXCEPT**
A. increasing specialization
B. expanding technology
C. governmental programs
D. financial pressures
E. lack of practice opportunities

638. The largest health service system operating under a unified management structure is represented by which of the following?
A. The Indian Health Service hospitals
B. The county hospitals
C. The public authority hospitals
D. The Veterans Administration hospitals
E. The church-related hospitals

639. The most costly component of long-term care is
A. mental health services
B. skilled nursing services
C. nursing home services
D. home health care services
E. rehabilitation services

640. The health care component identified as the largest user of the health care dollar in the United States is
A. physicians
B. hospitals
C. research
D. drugs
E. supplies

**641.** The largest payer of medical care expenses is
   A. private health insurance
   B. individuals
   C. employers
   D. government
   E. unions

**642.** Managed care plans include each of the following **EXCEPT**
   A. health maintenance organizations (HMO)
   B. independent practice associations (IPA)
   C. preferred provider organizations (PPO)
   D. exclusive provider organizations (EPO)
   E. group medical practices (GMP)

**643.** The predominant mode of physician reimbursement in 1992 was
   A. salary
   B. capitation
   C. fee for service
   D. point of service
   E. contracted care

**Questions 644–646:**
Choose the best match.

   A. independent practice association or open-model health maintenance organization
   B. closed panel or staff-model health maintenance organization
   C. preferred provider organization

**644.** The plan contracts with or directly hires providers who care exclusively for enrollees

**645.** The plan contracts with community-based providers, who are not exclusively bound to enrollees

**646.** The plan negotiates with community-based providers to obtain discounted fees

**Questions 647–649:**
Choose the best match.

    **A.** Medicare
    **B.** Medicaid
    **C.** Supplemental Security Income

**647.** A joint federal and state program that may cover the medically needy and the categorically needy

**648.** A federal program whose eligibility includes persons aged 65 years and older and people with end-stage renal disease

**649.** A federal program whose eligibility includes the blind, aged, and those who receive aid to families with dependent children

**650.** Important health indicators used to assess the status of maternal and child health include all of the following **EXCEPT**
    **A.** maternal mortality rates
    **B.** fertility rates
    **C.** pregnancy outcomes
    **D.** contraceptive use rates
    **E.** birth rates

**651.** When assessing factors associated with pregnancy outcome, the most precise measure is
    **A.** infant mortality rates
    **B.** infant birth and death rates
    **C.** maternal mortality rates
    **D.** fertility rates and birth rates
    **E.** infant birth rates

**652.** Social and demographic changes contributing to the health problems of women and children in the United States include all of the following **EXCEPT**
    **A.** increase in the number of mothers in the work force
    **B.** increase in the number of marriages ending in divorce
    **C.** increase in the number of homeless mothers and children
    **D.** decreased availability of health care
    **E.** increase in number of children living in poverty

**653.** When reviewing world infant mortality rates, the United States ranks closest to
   **A.** first
   **B.** tenth
   **C.** twentieth
   **D.** fortieth
   **E.** fiftieth

**654.** Social trends adversely affecting maternal and child health services include all of the following **EXCEPT**
   **A.** family planning methods
   **B.** malpractice crisis
   **C.** sexual abuse within families
   **D.** HIV infection rates
   **E.** new drugs of abuse

**655.** The goals of maternal and child health services include all of the following **EXCEPT**
   **A.** promoting healthy relationships within the family
   **B.** encouraging desired pregnancies
   **C.** providnig early intervention in the health problems of women and children
   **D.** monitoring school attendance
   **E.** reducing the risk for adult diseases

**656.** Health planning may focus on achieving changes in each of the following **EXCEPT**
   **A.** the characteristics of individuals
   **B.** demographics of the community
   **C.** the social aspects of the environment
   **D.** economic and legal factors
   **E.** organizational objectives

**657.** The nation's first major health services program was the
   **A.** comprehensive health planning program
   **B.** Hill-Burton program
   **C.** health maintenance legislation
   **D.** regional medical program
   **E.** American Red Cross

**658.** The most common type of health care planning used in the United States is
A. institution-based planning
B. program planning
C. population-based planning
D. agency planning
E. community planning

**659.** A health benefit associated with the use of oral contraceptives is
A. protection against both endometrial and ovarian cancer
B. protection against cervical cancer
C. protection against liver tumors
D. protection against bone cancer
E. protection against breast cancer

**660.** Risks associated with oral contraceptive use include
A. myocardial infarction and stroke
B. pelvic inflammatory disease
C. iron deficiency anemia
D. ectopic pregnancy
E. endometrial cancer

**661.** Family planning programs may improve health by all of the following **EXCEPT**
A. permitting a couple to choose the number and spacing of their children
B. permitting a woman to delay childbearing until her 30s and 40s
C. playing a role in decreasing the transmission of HIV
D. increasing divorce rates
E. allowing closer parent-child interaction

**662.** The primary goal of the national family planning program in the United States is to
A. reduce population growth
B. prevent unintended pregnancies
C. improve the health of women and children
D. regulate child spacing
E. improve pregnancy outcomes

**Questions 663–665:**
Match.

    **A.** health protection
    **B.** health promotion
    **C.** preventive health services

**663.** Smoking cessation, improved nutrition, alcohol and drug abuse reduction

**664.** Family planning, high blood pressure control, and immunizations

**665.** Accidental injury control, community water supply fluoridation, occupational health and safety

**666.** The three major foci for *Healthy People 2000,* a set of national priorities for public health, are
    **A.** access, equity, and comparison
    **B.** access, protection, and prevention
    **C.** protection, prevention, and promotion
    **D.** education, primary care, and rehabilitation
    **E.** managed care, cost effectiveness, and equal access

**667.** The most prevalent form of contraception in the world
    **A.** rhythm and fertility awareness
    **B.** surgical sterilization
    **C.** intrauterine devices
    **D.** oral contraceptives
    **E.** barrier devices

**668.** On a worldwide scale, the most births are prevented by which of the following methods?
    **A.** Rhythm and fertility awareness
    **B.** Surgical sterilization
    **C.** Breast-feeding
    **D.** Oral contraceptives
    **E.** Barrier devices

**669.** When compared with other nations, the teenage pregnancy rate in the United States is
   A. among the lowest
   B. among the highest
   C. comparable to other western countries
   D. comparable to developing nations
   E. steadily decreasing

**670.** Public health problems associated with prisons and jails include all of the following **EXCEPT**
   A. substance abuse, alcohol, and drugs
   B. AIDS, hepatitis, and venereal disease
   C. mental illness and suicide
   D. tuberculosis
   E. heart disease and stress

**Questions 671–676:**
Match the responsibilities with each organization.

   A. oversees the science of preventive medicine through basic science and applied research
   B. conducts research into the treatment of major categories of disease
   C. provides funds for clinical services for the poor, aged, and totally disabled
   D. provides services to indigenous populations
   E. evaluates the safety of food and drugs
   F. conducts its public health functions through a group of technically oriented branches

**671.** Health Care Financing Administration (HCFA)

**672.** Public Health Service (PHS)

**673.** Food and Drug Administration (FDA)

**674.** Centers for Disease Control and Prevention (CDC)

**675.** Indian Health Services (IHS)

**676.** National Institutes of Health (NIH)

**677.** Characteristics of international tobacco use include all of the following **EXCEPT**

**A.** the use of cigarettes being equated with economic and social success

**B.** tobacco becoming established as a cash crop, displacing subsistence agriculture

**C.** tobacco advertising and promotion being frequently less restricted than in the United States

**D.** smoking rates being still low compared to the United States

**E.** government revenue from tobacco growing and processing becoming an important tax base

**678.** Major international health problems associated with industrial development include all of the following **EXCEPT**

**A.** the use of infant formula rather than breast milk

**B.** the use of tobacco products

**C.** the cost of health care

**D.** environmental pollution

**E.** the increased use of automobiles

**679.** The traditional health problems of developing countries arise primarily from each of the following **EXCEPT**

**A.** infectious diseases

**B.** maldistribution of health care workers

**C.** uncontrolled population growth

**D.** poor immunization coverage

**E.** malnutrition

**680.** The worldwide rate of human population growth has changed from linear to exponential in growth for all of the following reasons **EXCEPT**

**A.** improved nutrition resulting from changes in climatic conditions

**B.** reduced risks of infant death from infections resulting from ecologic changes

**C.** treatment of infectious disease by antibiotics

**D.** changes in attitudes toward family size that influence traditional methods used to limit the number of offspring

**E.** improved nutrition as a result of increased areas of agriculture

**681.** The high incidence of significant respiratory-borne diseases among recruits in military training camps comes from each of the following organisms **EXCEPT**
A. adenoviruses type 4
B. rhinovirus
C. streptococci
D. adenovirus type 7
E. meningococci

**682.** Respiratory-borne diseases among recruits in military training camps are due to all of the following **EXCEPT**
A. person-to-person spread
B. bacterial agents
C. living conditions that permit close contact
D. viral agents
E. low immunization rates

**683.** Factors shaping health policy in the United States include all of the following **EXCEPT**
A. the character of the American people
B. the concept of federalism
C. the concept of pluralism
D. the concept of socialism
E. the concept of incrementalism

**684.** Power centers in the health care field that most influence the nature of health care and the role of government include all of the following **EXCEPT**
A. medical schools
B. insurance companies
C. special interest groups
D. hospitals
E. physicians

**685.** In the importance of their effects on humans, the most destructive natural disasters are
A. earthquakes
B. storms and floods
C. ecologic disasters
D. volcanoes
E. tsunamis

**686.** Whether measured by economic loss or by death and injuries, the geographic area most susceptible to natural disasters is
  A. Latin America and Africa
  B. North America, Europe, and Australia
  C. Asia
  D. South America
  E. Europe and Australia

**Questions 687–690:**
Match the following.

  A. industrial accidents
  B. fires, explosions, crashes, and spills
  C. earthquakes and volcanic eruptions
  D. flash floods and coastal and river floods

**687.** Climatologic disasters

**688.** Geologic disasters

**689.** Catastrophic events

**690.** Sudden chemical exposures

**691.** Key public health responses to mitigate disaster consequences include all of the following **EXCEPT**
  A. stringent building codes and land management
  B. education of public
  C. an early warning system
  D. certification of fatalities
  E. preparation of relief plans

**692.** The dominant ethical principle of public health is
  A. respect for autonomy
  B. beneficence
  C. nonmaleficence
  D. justice
  E. equality

**693.** The most effective means of temporary contraception that a woman can use is
- **A.** intrauterine devices
- **B.** oral contraception (the pill)
- **C.** spermatocidal jelly
- **D.** diaphragm
- **E.** condom

**694.** Of the following, which is not a contraindication for using oral contraceptives?
- **A.** coronary artery disease
- **B.** stroke
- **C.** breast-feeding an infant over 6 weeks of age
- **D.** pregnancy
- **E.** impaired liver function

**695.** Concerning intrauterine devices (IUD) as a means of contraception, identify the **INCORRECT** statement.
- **A.** IUD users have about half the risk of unintended pregnancies as those relying on the condom
- **B.** Wearing an IUD is absolutely contraindicated for women with active pelvic infection
- **C.** Use of an IUD is contraindicated in those with uterine or cervical malignancy
- **D.** Mortality rate for IUD users is about 3 per million per year
- **E.** Uterine perforation is less likely to occur when an IUD is inserted into the uterus of a lactating woman

**696.** Concerning sterilization of both men and women, identify the **INCORRECT** statement.
- **A.** Voluntary surgical sterilization is followed by about 0.4 unintended pregnancies per 100 procedures in the first year after surgery
- **B.** Long-term adverse health effects associated with vasectomy continue to be of serious concern
- **C.** China and India exceed the United States (and probably the rest of the world) in the number of surgical sterilizations
- **D.** Human studies have failed to confirm a serious risk of atherosclerosis in men who have undergone vasectomy
- **E.** Globally almost 100 million couples are reported to be using sterilization as a form of fertility control

**697.** The tendency for the number of births in a population to continue increasing despite a fertility decline is referred to as
   **A.** crude birth rate
   **B.** population momentum
   **C.** fecundity phenomenon
   **D.** fertility gap
   **E.** population retardation

**698.** Recent US data concerning teenage pregnancy and fertility reveal which of the following to be true?
   **A.** Decreasing proportions of unmarried teens having sexual intercourse
   **B.** Decrease in premarital conceptions
   **C.** Decreased contraceptive use
   **D.** Increased abortion among first premarital pregnancies
   **E.** Increased legitimization of births through marriage

**699.** Concerning death rates by race, sex, and age for United States in 1985, identify the **INCORRECT** statement.
   **A.** White women had the lowest estimated age-adjusted death rate
   **B.** Black women had the second lowest age-adjusted death rate
   **C.** Black men had the highest age-adjusted death rate
   **D.** White men had age-adjusted death rates that were worse than black women but better than black men
   **E.** There was little or no difference between the age-adjusted or crude death rates of any of these four groups

**700.** Fluoridation of water is a method of
   **A.** decreasing bacterial population
   **B.** preventing growth of bacteria
   **C.** preventing bacterial toxin formation
   **D.** limiting multiplication of viruses
   **E.** preventing dental decay

**701.** The leading cause of maternal deaths in the United States is
   **A.** toxemia
   **B.** hemorrhage
   **C.** sepsis
   **D.** respiratory complications
   **E.** cardiovascular complications

**702.** All of the following disorders are believed to be solely the result of genetic factors **EXCEPT**
A. epilepsy
B. hemophilia
C. fibrocystic disease of the pancreas
D. multiple polyposis of the colon
E. xeroderma pigmentosum

**703.** All of the following are minimum functions of a state health department as defined by the American Public Health Association **EXCEPT**
A. the study of state health problems and planning for their solution
B. coordination and technical supervision of local health activities
C. financial aid to local health departments
D. the enactment of sanitary regulations applicable in local health departments
E. the establishment of maximum standards for local health work

**704.** The state health department is responsible for the protection of the general health and welfare of the citizens of that state. The supervision of these activities is usually carried out by the
A. governor of the state
B. state board of health
C. commissioner or director of health
D. state public health association
E. directors of health planning agencies

**Questions 705–707:**
Select the *one* lettered item that is most closely associated with the question. Each lettered heading may be selected once, more than once, or not at all.

A. fertility
B. fecundity
C. crude birth rate (CBR)
D. total fertility rate

**705.** The ability to produce live-born young

**706.** Number of live births per 1000 population during a year

**707.** Provides a single number to summarize the fertility level

# Health Care Organization

## Answers and Discussion

**633. (E)** A solid understanding of the system is essential for all participants: provider, consumer, payer, and policy maker. (**Ref. 2,** p. 1065)

**634. (D)** An aging population and a growing proportion of minorities influences the location and types of services that need to be provided. The change from infectious to chronic diseases; technologic advances; and legal issues, including malpractice concerns, have also been important. (**Ref. 2,** p. 1065)

**635. (A)** Disease of the heart was among the top five leading causes of death identified both in 1900 and 1985. In the early 1900s the leading causes of death were infectious diseases. In 1985, the major causes of death were the chronic diseases of an aging population. (**Ref. 2,** pp. 1065, 1066)

**636. (C)** There are three competing sources of authority in the hospital: the governing board, the administration, and the medical staff. The governing board has the ultimate responsibility for the hospital. (**Ref. 2,** p. 1068)

**637. (E)** Developments in medical practice, especially increasing specialization and expansion of technology, have spurred the group practice movement. Changing lifestyles, the cost of establishing a practice, external pressures on practitioners, and governmental programs have also affected the traditional dominance of solo practice. (**Ref. 2,** p. 1070)

**638.** (**D**)  The Veterans Administration is the largest health service system under a unified management structure in the United States. (**Ref. 2,** p. 1071)

**639.** (**C**)  The nursing home is the most costly component of long-term care. Financial support for nursing home care generally is inadequate to provide the level of services, activities, physical environment, and staff required. (**Ref. 2,** p. 1071)

**640.** (**B**)  The hospital is the largest user of health care dollars. Although physicians account for under 20% of expenditures directly, they control many other resources. (**Ref. 2,** p. 1074)

**641.** (**D**)  The largest payer of medical care expenses is government (about 40%), with private health insurance close behind (about 33%). (**Ref. 2,** p. 1074)

**642.** (**E**)  New insurance approaches include managed care plans. Managed care systems include all options mentioned, plus a growing number of variations. (**Ref. 2,** p. 1077)

**643.** (**C**)  Physicians can be reimbursed through three mechanisms: fee for service, capitation, and salary. The predominant mode of reimbursement in this country is fee for service, where a physician renders care and the patient or third party reimburses the physician on a per-service basis. (**Ref. 2,** p. 1074)

**644.** (**B**); **645.** (**A**); **646.** (**C**)  In the staff model HMO, the plan contracts with or directly hires providers who care exclusively for enrollees in the plan. The independent practice association (or open-model or foundation HMO) contracts with community-based providers who are not exclusively bound to the enrollees in the plan and who care for other patients as well. In a preferred provider organization (PPO), the plan negotiates with the community-based providers to obtain discounted fees. (**Ref. 2,** p. 1077)

**647.** (**B**); **648.** (**A**); **649.** (**C**)  Medicaid is a joint federal-state program. The states administer and jointly fund Medicaid programs and agree to provide a minimum set of services. The federal government requires that these services be provided to the categorically needy, a determination based on income. Medicare is a federal program with two parts: A and B. Medicare eligibility generally includes those people aged 65 years and over, the permanently and totally disabled, and people with end-stage renal disease. The categorically needy are people who receive cash payments under the Supplemental Security Income (SSI-welfare payments) program. These people include those who are blind, those who are permanently and totally disabled, the aged, and those who receive aid to families with dependent children. (**Ref. 2,** p. 1077)

**650.** (**D**)   Maternal mortality rates have reached such a low level in the United States that they are less valuable now. Maternal health is reflected in fertility rates and birth rates as well as pregnancy-related morbidity and mortality rates. Pregnancy outcomes have become a more important measure of maternal health and quality of maternity services provided. (**Ref. 2,** p. 1095)

**651.** (**B**)   Infant mortality rate remains an important though crude measure of maternal child health. Linking infant birth and death records has provided a more precise way of assessing factors associated with pregnancy outcome. (**Ref. 2,** p. 1095)

**652.** (**D**)   Social and demographic changes are important indicators of the status of mothers and children. Over the last 20 years there have been increases in the percentage of mothers in the work force, the percentage of marriages that end in divorce, the numbers of homeless mothers and children, and the percentage of children living in poverty. These social problems contribute directly or indirectly to most of the health problems of women and children. (**Ref. 2,** p. 1096)

**653.** (**C**)   In infant mortality rates, the United States ranks twentieth in the world, a fact that many attribute at least in part to the inadequate provision of maternal and infant services. (**Ref. 2,** p. 1096)

**654.** (**A**)   Social trends of the last decade having an effect on maternal and child health services include the malpractice crisis, preconceptual health promotion, prenatal care, the spread of human immunodeficiency virus infection, sexual abuse, and new drugs of abuse. (**Ref. 2,** p. 1096)

**655.** **(D)** The goals of maternal child health services are to encourage desired pregnancy, to promote healthy relationships within the family, to optimize the normal developmental processes to allow the child to achieve his or her fullest potential, to prevent child health problems and reduce the risks of adult health problems, and to provide early intervention in the health problems of women and children so as to minimize morbidity and mortality in a cost-effective manner. (**Ref. 2,** p. 1096)

**656.** **(B)** Health planning may focus on achieving changes in the characteristics of individuals, in the characteristics of organizations, or in the physical, economic, legal, and social characteristics of the environment. (**Ref. 2,** p. 1079)

**657.** **(B)** Concerns over the health status of the population, the maldistribution of hospitals, and the poor condition of most hospitals prompted the federal government to establish the nation's first major health services planning and construction subsidy program, the Hill-Burton Program (the Hospital Survey and Construction Act of 1946). (**Ref. 2,** p. 1080)

**658.** **(B)** Health care planning is designated as population-based, institution-based, and program planning. Program planning is the most common type of planning being done in the United States and incorporates features of population-based and institution-based planning. (**Ref. 2,** p. 1081)

**659.** **(A)** Documented noncontraceptive health benefits associated with the use of oral contraceptives include protection against both endometrial and ovarian cancer. (**Ref. 2,** p. 1102)

**660.** **(A)** Oral contraceptive use has been clearly associated with an increased risk of myocardial infarction, venous thrombosis, and stroke. (**Ref. 2,** p. 1102)

**661.** **(D)** Family planning programs may influence health by permitting a woman to bear children at an age when the risk of health problems to her and her offspring is lowest and by permitting a couple to choose the number of children and determine the spacing of their children. Family planning also plays a key role in preventing AIDS because of its relation to both heterosexual and mother-to-infant transmission of HIV. (**Ref. 2,** pp. 1106, 1108)

**662. (B)** The goal of the national family planning program in the United States seeks primarily to prevent unintended pregnancies. (**Ref. 2,** p. 1100)

**663. (B); 664. (C); 665. (A)** Health promotion is among the health strategy targets associated with the year 2000 goals. Goals associated with health promotion for population groups include smoking cessation, alcohol and drug abuse reduction, improved nutrition, exercise and fitness, and stress control. Goals associated with preventive health services for individuals include family planning, pregnancy and infant care, immunizations, sexually transmissible diseases services, and high blood pressure control. Goals associated with health protection for population groups include toxic agent control, occupational health and safety, accidental injury control, community water supply fluoridation, and infectious agent control. (**Ref. 2,** p. 1116)

**666. (C)** The 1990 goals, the National Health Objectives, defined a set of national priorities for public health. The goals are grouped into three major foci: prevention, protection, and promotion. (**Ref. 2,** p. 1116)

**667. (B)** Surgical sterilization is estimated to be the most prevalent form of contraception in the world today. Globally more than 100 million couples are using this form of birth control; an estimated 95 million women have undergone tubal sterilization, making it the most widely used contraceptive method in the world. (**Ref. 2,** p. 1104)

**668. (C)** It is asserted that on a worldwide scale, more births are prevented by breast feeding than by any other method of contraception. (**Ref. 2,** p. 1104)

**669. (B)** Compared with other nations for which data are available on teenage pregnancy, the United States has a rate (95/1000) that is among the highest. (**Ref. 2,** p. 1108)

**670. (E)** Significant public health problems that are concentrated in American correctional facilities include substance abuse, AIDS, hepatitis, trauma, violence, tuberculosis, suicide, mental illness, and venereal disease. **(Ref. 2,** p. 1160)

**671. (C); 672. (F); 673. (E); 674. (A); 675. (D); 676. (B)** National programs were developed by the federal government to promote specific policies. Health services are provided by two major branches of the Department of Health and Human Services (DHHS). One function of the DHHS is to provide funds for clinical services for the poor, the aged, and the totally disabled through the Health Care Financing Administration (HCFA). The other major branch for health services is the Public Health Service (PHS). The PHS carries out its public health functions through a group of technically oriented branches. It is responsible for evaluation of safe food and drugs through the Food and Drug Administration (FDA), the science of preventive medicine through basic and applied research in the Centers for Disease Control and Prevention (CDC), for services to indigenous populations (native Indians and Eskimos) through the Indian Health Services (IHS), and research into treatment of major categories of diseases through the National Institutes of Health (NIH). **(Ref. 2,** p. 1114)

**677. (D)** Adoption of cigarette smoking, often without the restraining laws and regulations of the affluent industrial nations, is causing serious problems for developing nations. The tobacco companies are able to promote and advertise their product without restraint. Also, the use of cigarettes is equated with social and economic success, and tobacco has become established as a cash crop, displacing needed subsistence agriculture. **(Ref. 2,** p. 1136)

**678. (C)** International health problems associated with industrial development include the adoption of cigarette smoking, an increase in traffic injury and premature death associated with the influx of automobiles, the persuasion to use infant formula rather than breast milk, and environmental pollution from poor industrial standards. **(Ref. 2,** p. 1136)

**679. (D)** The traditional health problems of the developing world arise from the interaction of three forces: infectious diseases, malnutrition, and uncontrolled population growth. **(Ref. 2,** p. 1132)

**680. (C)** Demographers believe that increases in the world's population result from improved nutrition, changes in climatic conditions, and the opening up to agriculture of vast areas in the Americas and Australia, reduced risks of infant death from infections resulting from ecologic changes, and subtle changes in attitudes toward family size that influenced traditional methods used to limit the numbers of offspring. (**Ref. 2**, p. 1131)

**681. (B)** The respiratory-borne diseases of primary importance in military recruit camps have included acute respiratory diseases due to adenoviruses types 4 and 7, meningococcal disease, and streptococcal disease. (**Ref. 2**, p. 1147)

**682. (E)** The high incidence of respiratory-borne diseases among recruits in military training camps is the result of person-to-person spread of a number of viral and bacterial agents among susceptibles assembled under barracks living conditions that permit frequent close contact. (**Ref. 2**, p. 1147)

**683. (D)** Special factors that shape public policy in the United States include the American character, federalism, pluralism, and incrementalism. (**Ref. 2**, pp. 1166, 1168)

**684. (A)** Four power centers in the health care field that influence the nature of health care and the role of government are: hospitals, large insurance organizations, physicians, and a highly diversified group of participants in profit-making activities within the health care arena. (**Ref. 2**, p. 1168)

**685. (B)** In approximate order of the importance of their effects on humans, the most destructive natural disasters are climatologic (ie, floods, storms) rather than geologic (ie, earthquakes, volcanic eruptions, and tsunamis). (**Ref. 2**, p. 1173)

**686. (C)** Asia is most prone to natural disasters; Latin America and Africa are intermediate; and North America, Europe, and Australia are least prone. (**Ref. 2**, p. 1173)

**687. (D); 688. (C); 689. (B); 690. (A)** Sudden disasters are classified as climatologic and geologic disasters, catastrophic events, and sudden chemical and radiation exposures. Climatologic disasters include flash floods, storms, and more predictable coastal and river floods. Geologic disasters include earthquakes and volcanic eruptions. Catastrophic events include fires, explosions, crashes, and spills, with or without the release of toxic materials. Industrial accidents are an important source of sudden chemical exposure. **(Ref. 2, p. 1174)**

**691. (D)** Secondary prevention measures designed to mitigate disaster consequences include land use and building codes, public education, early warning systems, and preparation of relief plans. **(Ref. 2, p. 1180)**

**692. (B)** The dominant ethical principle for public health is beneficence. The aim of public health services should be to enlighten people about risks to health and to assist people in gaining greater control over environmental, social, and other conditions that influence their own health. **(Ref. 2, p. 1194)**

**693. (B)** Oral contraception (the pill) is the most effective means of temporary contraception. National survey data show that the pill has a failure rate of 2.4 unintended pregnancies per 100 married sexually active women during the first year of use. The risk of pregnancy for women who use oral contraception is half that of women who use IUDs. An estimated 10,000,000 women in the United States used oral contraceptives in 1982. It is the most popular method of birth control for women younger than 30 years of age. **(Ref. 2, p. 1102)**

**694. (C)** Estrogen-containing contraceptive pills are not prescribed for women during the first 6 weeks that they are breast-feeding an infant. Other contraindications for the pill are unexplained vaginal bleeding, pregnancy, stroke, hypertension, gallbladder disease, diabetes, plans for surgery within four weeks of taking the pill, and injury or embolization of the legs. The risk of problems increases with cigarette smoking, age, and the use of pills that have a high estrogen content. **(Ref. 2, pp. 1102, 1103)**

**695. (E)** It is more likely to occur if insertion takes place during lactation. Three conditions—pelvic inflammatory disease, uterine perforation, and second trimester septic spontaneous abortion—account for virtually all of the hospitalizations in users of IUDs. (**Ref. 2,** p. 1103)

**696.** **(B)** Long-term adverse health effects associated with vasectomy are not of the serious concern they once were, because human studies have failed to confirm animal studies. Sterilized monkeys who were fed high-cholesterol diets showed more serious atherosclerosis than those monkeys that had not been sterilized. China reported about 36 million sterilizations in 1980 and India about 23 million. (**Ref. 2,** p. 1106)

**697.** **(B)** The tendency for the number of births in a population to continue increasing even after a fertility decline has set in is referred to as population momentum. If a population has been growing at 2.5% per year with a constant crude birth rate for a long time, its number of births was increasing at 2.5 per year. Thus, if mortality rates stay relatively constant, the number of persons reaching age 15 will continue to increase at 2.5% for 15 years into the future no matter what happens to fertility rates in the meantime. The implications for developing countries are obvious, for no matter how rapidly fertility rates decline to replacement levels, these countries still have many years of rapid population growth ahead. (**Ref. 2,** pp. 1106, 1107)

**698.** **(D)** Increased abortion among first premarital pregnancies is true. All of the other answers are false. There is, however, an increase in the proportion of unmarried teens keeping their child once it is born. These facts raise questions about the adequacy of current sex education and family planning services for teenagers and about changing social patterns among teens. (**Ref. 2,** p. 1008)

**699.** **(E)** The differences were as follows:

White women:  390 deaths/100,000 population

Black women:  585 deaths/100,000 population

White men:  690 deaths/100,000 population

Black men:  1029 deaths/100,000 population

(Figures are rounded for simplicity) (**Ref. 92,** p. 6)

**700. (E)** Fluoridation of municipal water supplies is a common practice to prevent dental caries. A fluoride ion level of 0.6 to 1.2 mg/L (depending on temperature) will prevent dental caries with no mottling of enamel. (**Ref. 2,** p. 1008)

**701. (A)** Regarding all causes of death, toxemia leads the list for maternal mortality. Maternal mortality runs less than 400 deaths per year in the United States. (**Ref. 93,** p. 463)

**702. (A)** Epilepsy appears to involve complex interactions (as yet unanalyzed) between genetic and nongenetic causal factors. (**Ref. 94,** p. 323)

**703. (E)** The state health department is required to establish minimal, not maximal, standards for local health work. The other functions are: the maintenance of central and branch laboratory services, including diagnostic, sanitary, chemical, biologic, and research activities; the collection, tabulation, and analysis of vital statistics; the collection and distribution of information concerning preventable disease; the maintenance of a safe quality of water and the control of waste disposal; establishment and maintenance of minimal standards of milk sanitation; provision of service to aid industry in the control of occupational hazards; the establishment of qualifications for health personnel; and formulation of plans in cooperation with other organizations for meeting all health needs. (**Ref. 95**)

**704. (C)** The commissioner or director of health is the administrative head of the state health activities. His or her line of authority is usually from the governor, with the state board of health service serving as an advisory board. (**Ref. 95**)

**705. (B); 706. (C); 707. (D)** Fecundity is the ability to produce. It is difficult to measure, since it refers to the theoretical ability of a woman or couple to conceive and carry a fetus to term. Crude birth rate can be shown as follows:

$$CBR = \frac{\text{live births in 1 year}}{\text{midyear population}} \times 1000 \text{ live-born young}$$

Total fertility rate is the sum of the age-specific fertility rates and provides a simple index of the fertility level. (**Ref. 2,** pp. 44, 45)

# References

1. Fisher M, ed. *Guide to Clinical Preventive Services* (Report of the US Preventive Services Task Force). Baltimore, Md: Williams & Wilkins; 1989.

2. Last JM, Wallace RB, eds. *Maxcy-Rosenau-Last Public Health and Preventive Medicine.* 13th ed. Norwalk, Conn: Appleton & Lange; 1992.

3. Morgan JW. *Concise Epidemiology.* 3rd ed. Bryn Mawr, Calif: MDM Consulting; 1994.

4. McGinnis MJ, ed. *The Clinician's Handbook of Preventive Services.* Washington, DC: Public Health Service, Office of Disease Prevention and Health Promotion; 1994; U.S. Department of Health and Human Services, publication #8507-7.

5. Nadakavukaren A. *Our Global Environment, a Health Perspective.* 4th ed. Prospect Heights, Ill: Waveland Press, Inc; 1995.

6. Centers for Disease Control. *MMWR Morb Mortal Wkly Rep.* 1994; 43:RR-7.

7. Centers for Disease Control. *MMWR Morb Mortal Wkly Rep.* 1994; 43:31.

8. Greenberg RS, et al. *Medical Epidemiology.* Norwalk, Conn: Appleton & Lange; 1993.

9. Kramer MS. *Clinical Epidemiology and Biostatistics.* New York, NY: Springer-Verlag; 1988.

10. Lilienfeld AM, Lilienfeld DE. *Foundations of Epidemiology.* 2nd ed. New York, NY: Oxford University Press; 1980.

11. Rothman KJ. *Modern Epidemiology.* Boston, Mass: Little, Brown & Co Inc; 1986.

12. Breslow NE, Day NE. *Statistical Methods in Cancer Research, The Analysis of Case–Control Studies.* Lyon, France: IARC Publications; 1980; 84–121.

13. Kuzma J. *Basic Statistics for the Health Sciences.* Moutain View, Calif: Mayfield Publishing Co; 1984.

14. Mausner JS, Borhn K. *Epidemiology, An Introductory Text.* Philadelphia, Pa: WB Saunders Co; 1985.

15. Clark DW, Macmahon B. *Preventive Medicine.* 2nd ed. Boston, Mass: Little, Brown & Co Inc; 1980.

16. Arnon SS, Midura TF, Clay SA, et al. Intestinal infection and toxin production by *Clostridium botulinum* as one cause of sudden infant death syndrome. *Lancet.* 1978;41:1273–1276.

17. *Guide for Adult Immunization.* 2nd ed. Philadelphia, Pa: American College of Physicians; 1990.

18. *Heart Facts.* Dallas, Texas: American Heart Association; 1987.

19. Benenson AS, ed. *Control of Communicable Diseases in Man.* 15th ed. Washington, DC: American Public Health Association; 1990.

20. Berkow RB, Fletcher AJ, eds. *The Merck Manual of Diagnosis and Therapy.* 15th ed. Rahway, NJ: Merck, Sharp & Dohme Research Laboratories; 1987.

21. Bloch AB, Cauthen GM, Onorato IM, et al. Nationwide survey of drug-resistant tuberculosis in the United States. *JAMA.* 1994; 27:665–671.

22. Brauwald E, Isselbacher KJ, Wilson JV. *Harrison's Principles of Internal Medicine.* 13th ed. New York, NY: McGraw-Hill Inc; 1994.

23. *CA: Cancer Clin.* 1991;41.

24. Centers for Disease Control. *Health Information for International Travel.* Atlanta, Ga: Centers for Disease Control; 1993. US Dept of Health and Human Services publication 93-8280.

25. Centers for Disease Control. *HIV/AIDS Surveillance Report.* July, 1991.

26. Centers for Disease Control. *MMWR Morb Mortal Wkly Rep.* 1991;40:RR-12:59.

27. Centers for Disease Control. *MMWR Morb Mortal Wkly Rep.* 1989;38:205, 219.

28. Centers for Disease Control. *MMWR Morb Mortal Wkly Rep.* 1992;41:RR-17.

29. Centers for Disease Control. *MMWR Morb Mortal Wkly Rep.* 1994;43:155.

30. Centers for Disease Control. *MMWR Morb Mortal Wkly Rep.* 1995;44:387.

31. Centers for Disease Control. *MMWR Morb Mortal Wkly Rep.* 1995;44:381.

32. Centers for Disease Control. *MMWR Morb Mortal Wkly Rep.* 1992;41:RR-17:1.

33. Centers for Disease Control. *MMWR Morb Mortal Wkly Rep.* 1982;31:35.

34. Centers for Disease Control. *MMWR Morb Mortal Wkly Rep.* 1991;40:RR-4.

35. Centers for Disease Control. *MMWR Morb Mortal Wkly Rep.* 1991;40:25.

36. Centers for Disease Control. *MMWR Morb Mortal Wkly Rep.* 1989;38:21–24.

37. Centers for Disease Control. *MMWR Morb Mortal Wkly Rep.* 1991;40:RR-1.

38. Centers for Disease Control. *MMWR Morb Mortal Wkly Rep.* 1990;39:RR-2.

39. Centers for Disease Control. *MMWR Morb Mortal Wkly Rep.* 1991;40:22.

40. Centers for Disease Control. *MMWR Morb Mortal Wkly Rep.* 1990;39:36.

41. Centers for Disease Control. *MMWR Morb Mortal Wkly Rep.* 1989;38:RR-8.

42. Centers for Disease Control. *MMWR Morb Mortal Wkly Rep.* 1989;38:64–65.

43. Centers for Disease Control. *MMWR Morb Mortal Wkly Rep.* 1989;38:5.

44. Centers for Disease Control. *MMWR Morb Mortal Wkly Rep.* 1985;34:23.

45. Centers for Disease Control. *MMWR Morb Mortal Wkly Rep.* 1991;40:RR-6.

46. Centers for Disease Control. *MMWR Morb Mortal Wkly Rep.* 1989;38:13.

47. Centers for Disease Control. *MMWR Morb Mortal Wkly Rep.* 1982;31:35.

48. Centers for Disease Control. *MMWR Morb Mortal Wkly Rep.* 1986;35:30.

49. Centers for Disease Control. *MMWR Morb Mortal Wkly Rep.* 1986;35:34.

50. Centers for Disease Control. *MMWR Morb Mortal Wkly Rep.* 1986;35:1.

51. Centers for Disease Control. *MMWR Morb Mortal Wkly Rep.* 1991;40:32.

52. Centers for Disease Control. *MMWR Morb Mortal Wkly Rep.* 1990;38:51.

53. Centers for Disease Control. *MMWR Morb Mortal Wkly Rep.* 1990;38:1.

54. Centers for Disease Control. *MMWR Morb Mortal Wkly Rep.* 1991;40:RR-3.

55. Centers for Disease Control. *National Tuberculosis Training Initiative Core Curriculum on Tuberculosis.* New York, NY: American Thoracic Society; 1990.

56. Clark DW, McMahon B. *Preventive and Community Medicine.* 2nd ed. Boston, Mass: Little, Brown & Co Inc.; 1981.

57. Cole P, Morrison A. Basic issues in population screening for cancer. *J Nat Cancer Inst.* 1980;64:1263–1272.

58. Committee on Infectious Diseases. *Report of the Committee on Infectious Diseases.* 20th ed. Elk Grove Village, Ill: American Academy of Pediatrics; 1986.

59. Fishel S, Webster J, Jackson P, et al. Waterborne giardiasis in the United States 1965–84. *Lancet.* 1986;2:513–514.

60. Garner JS, Favero MS. *Guidelines for Handwashing and Hospital Environmental Control.* Atlanta, Ga: Centers for Disease Control; 1985. US Dept of Health, Education and Welfare publication #99-1117.

61. Goldman DA. Vancomycin resistant *Enterococcus faecium:* headline news. *Infec Control Hosp Epidemiol.* 1992; 13:695–699.

62. Hennekens CH, Buring, JE. *Epidemiology in Medicine.* Boston, Mass: Little, Brown & Co Inc; 1987.

63. Jawetz E, Melnick JL, Adelberg EA. *Review of Medical Microbiology.* 17th ed. Norwalk, Conn: Appleton & Lange; 1987.

64. Mandell GL, Douglas RG Jr, Bennett JE. *Principles and Practice of Infectious Disease.* 3rd ed. New York, NY: Churchill Livingston; 1990.

65. *Med Lett Drugs Ther.* 1990;32:21.

66. Nosten F, Luxemburger C, ter Kuile FO, et al. Treatment of multidrug-resistant *Plasmodium falciparum* malaria with 3-day artesunate-mefloquine combination. *J Infect Dis.* 1994;170: 971–977.

67. Steketee RW, Reid S, Cheng T, et al. Recurrent outbreaks of giardiasis in a child day care center, Wisconsin. *Am J of Public Health.* 1989;79:1–18.

68. Thompson R. *Travel and Routine Immunizations: A Practical Guide for the Medical Office.* Milwaukee, Wis: Shoreland Medical Marketing Inc; 1995.

69. *Foodborne Disease.* Washington, DC: US Department of Health, Education, and Welfare; September, 1985.

70. *The Surgeon General's Report on Nutrition and Health.* Washington, DC: US Public Health Service; 1988. US Depart of Health and Human Services publication 88-50210.

71. *Health Information for International Travel.* Atlanta, Ga: Centers for Disease Control; August, 1985. US Department of Health and Human Services publication (CDC)85-8280.

72. *Advisory Memorandum #88.* Washinton, DC: US Department of Health and Human Services; April 7, 1988.

73. US Preventive Services Task Force. *Guide to Clinical Preventive Services: An Assessment of the Effectiveness of 169 Interventions.* Baltimore, Md: Williams & Wilkins; 1989.

74. Woodley M, Whelan A. *The Washington Manual.* Boston, Mass: Little, Brown & Co Inc; 1992.

75. Centers for Disease Control. *MMWR Morb Mortal Wkly Rep.* 1985;34:22.

76. *Am Dent Assoc News.* 1994;25(10):12, 14.

77. Andreoli TE. *Cecil Essentials of Medicine.* 2nd ed. Philadelphia, Pa: WB Saunders Co; 1990.

78. Berkow R, Fletcher AJ, Chin B, eds. *The Merck Manual.* 15th ed. Rahway, NJ: Merck & Co; 1987.

79. Centers for Disease Control. *CDC Fact Book.* Washington, DC: US Dept of Health and Human Services; 1993.

80. Gilman AG. *Goodman and Gilman's the Pharmacological Basis of Therapeutics.* 8th ed. New York, NY: Macmillan Publishing Co; 1985.

81. Jakobiec A. *Principles and Practices of Ophthalmology.* Philadelphia, Pa: WB Saunders Co; 1994.

82. National Institutes of Health Consensus Conference, 1994: Helicobacter Pylori in PUD. *JAMA.* 1994;272:65–69.

83. Stone RM. *Pretest Assessment and Review: Harrison's Principles of Internal Medicine.* 12th ed. New York, NY: McGraw-Hill Inc; 1991.

84. US Institute of Medicine. *The Future of Public Health.* Washington, DC: National Academy Press; 1988.

85. Levy BS, Wegman DH. *Occupational Health.* Boston, Mass: Little, Brown & Co Inc; 1983.

86. Last JM, Wallace RB, eds. *Maxcy-Rosenau-Last Public Health and Preventive Medicine.* 13th ed. Norwalk, Conn: Appleton & Lange; 1992.

87. Jawetz E, Melnick JL, Adelberg EA. *Review of Medical Microbiology.* 17th ed. Norwalk, Conn: Appleton & Lange; 1987.

88. *CA: Cancer Clin.* 1985;35(1).

89. McGinnis MJ, ed. *The Clinician's Handbook of Preventive Services.* Washington, DC: Public Health Service, Office of Disease Prevention and Health Promotion; 1994; U.S. Department of Health and Human Services, publication #8507-7.

90. Brooks S. *Environmental Medicine.* St Louis, Mo: Mosby Year Book; 1995.

91. Levy BS, Wegman, DH, eds. *Occupational Health: Recognizing and Preventing Work-Related Disease.* 2nd ed. Boston, Mass: Little Brown & Co; 1988.

92. *Monthly Vital Stat Rep.* 1986;34:13.

93. Hanlon JJ, Pickett GE. *Public Health Administration and Practice.* 8th ed. St Louis, Mo: CV Mosby Co; 1984.

94. Leavell HR, Clark EG. *Preventive Medicine for the Doctor in His Community.* 3rd ed. New York, NY: McGraw-Hill Book Co, Inc; 1965.

95. US Institute of Medicine. *The Future of Public Health.* Washington, DC: National Academy Press; 1988.